Suzan

M000266018

Nature's Best
Heart
Medicine

New scientific discoveries reveal how flavonoids are beneficial for people with

- **Heart disease**
- **High blood pressure**
- **Varicose veins**
- **Circulation problems**
- **and more**

books Alive

Summertown
Tennessee

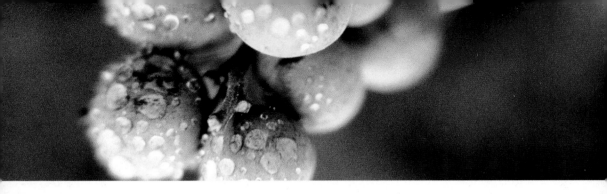

contents

Note: Conversions in this book (from imperial to metric) are not exact. They have been rounded to the nearest measurement for convenience. Exact measurements are given in imperial. The recipes in this book are by no means to be taken as therapeutic. They simply promote the philosophy of both the author and *alive* books in relation to whole foods, health, and nutrition, while incorporating the practical advice given by the author in the first section of the book.

Recipes

It is your constitutional right to educate yourself in health and medical knowledge, to seek helpful information and make use of it for your own benefit, and for that of your family. You are the one responsible for your health. In order to make decisions in all health matters, you must educate yourself. With this book and the guidance of a naturopath or alternative medical doctor, you will learn what is needed to achieve optimal health.

Those individuals currently taking pharmaceutical prescription drugs will want to talk to their health-care professional about the negative effects that the drugs can have on herbal remedies and nutritional supplements before combining them.

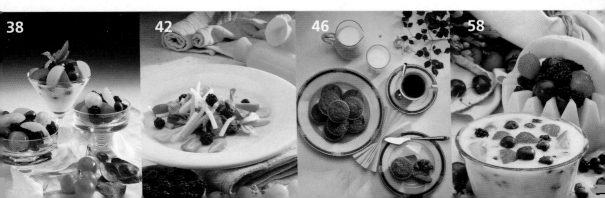

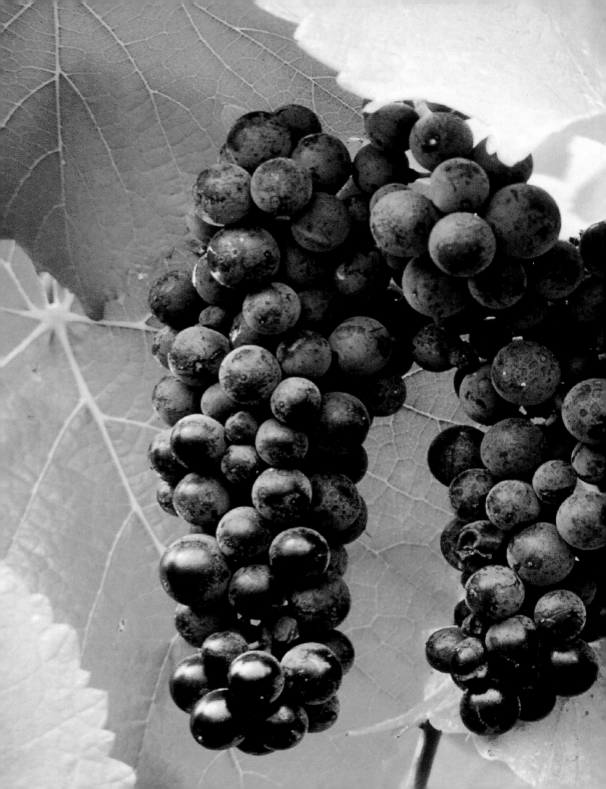

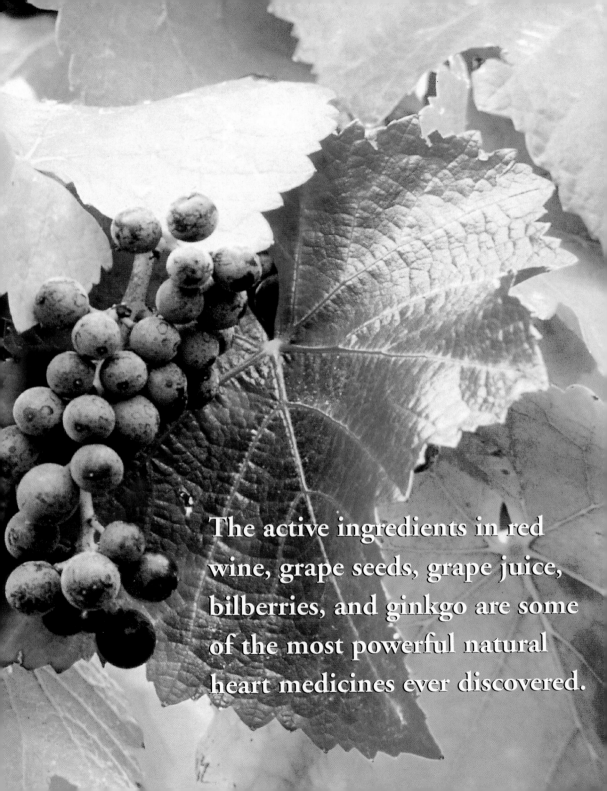

The active ingredients in red wine, grape seeds, grape juice, bilberries, and ginkgo are some of the most powerful natural heart medicines ever discovered.

Introduction . . . .

Heart disease is the number-one killer in our society. In fact, 40 percent of all deaths in North America are attributed to cardio-vascular disease. Prevention to most people means taking ASA daily. Heart disease is certainly not caused by a lack of Acetylsalicylic acid (ASA) in the bloodstream. The latest research suggests that along with other dietary and lifestyle factors, heart disease may be due to a lack of certain flavonoids in our diet.

Acetylsalicylic acid (ASA), is commonly prescribed to prevent heart disease, yet the side-effects kill too many people each year.

A particularly important set of flavonoids are plant colorings with differing chemical properties. They are found in berries, other fruits, seeds and barks. Our ancestors consumed much more of these flavonoids than we do today. According to a leading American heart specialist, flavonoids from grape seed extract, red wine extract, grape juice, and bilberries are better than ASA for preventing coronary artery disease.

Some researchers say that flavonoids are the best natural heart medicines yet discovered; these compounds, which give fruits and vegetables–especially berries–their bright colours, have been prescribed for their therapeutic benefits for more than a half a century in Europe. Since heart disease is the number one killer in our society, you need to know how to protect yourself against this preventable illness.

Flavonoids are special phytochemicals (plant nutrients) found everywhere in the plant kingdom. They include anthocyanin (anthos means flower and cyan means blue), catechin, hesperidin, pine bark extract, quercetin, and rutin. We will concentrate on anthocyanins, proanthocyanidins, and Oligomeric proanthocyanidins (OPCs).

Too many people die each year from the bleeding side effects of ASA. A recent study published in the British medical journal *The Lancet* showed that buffered or enteric-coated ASA tablets are not less harmful than plain ASA. The use of low doses of coated ASA carries a three-fold increased risk of major upper gastrointestinal bleeding. Other studies have shown that some individuals who take ASA daily to prevent coronary artery clot formation may not be well protected. So people may be suffering an increased risk of death from bleeding from an ASA a day all for nothing. In contrast, flavonoids come with no associated risks, only benefits. Flavonoids can even prevent the bleeding side-effects of ASA. A natural, safer alternative to ASA is willow bark tea or extract from health food stores.

How Berries and Seeds Support Heart Health

Two types of flavonoids, *anthocyanins and oligomeric proantho-cyanidins* (OPC), are powerful curative agents used by millions of people in Europe as natural "drugs" for improving circulation and strengthening the membranes of blood vessels and capillaries–that means improved heart health. Flavonoids can be used to treat these cardiovascular conditions:

- blood vessel weakness
- circulation disorders
- edema (water retention)
- inflammatory diseases
- varicose veins and other vein and artery disorders.

I know of one woman who had very bad circulation problems with her feet and had varicose veins–she often could not fit her feet into her shoes. I recommended that she start taking grapeseed OPC flavonoid supplements, and within a few weeks she said that she had not felt better for over ten years and that her feet had stopped swelling!

Beyond Heart Health

These substances are so valuable and versatile that they can treat much more than just your heart. Several clinical trials on bilberry (European blueberry) extract have documented the effective-ness of anthocyanin extracts for treating diabetic circulatory dis-eases and diabetic retinopathy. In France, OPCs from peanut skins and grape seed have been used to treat these conditions since the 1940s. Anthocyanins also enhance the structural integrity of artery walls; this could be crit-ical for preventing strokes. These

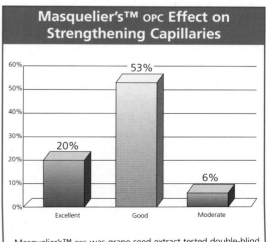

Masquelier's™ OPC Effect on Strengthening Capillaries

Masquelier's™ OPC was grape seed extract tested double-blind on a group of elderly people who had very fragile capillaries. Seventy-nine percent had noticeable improvement after two weeks with 100 to 150 mg per day.

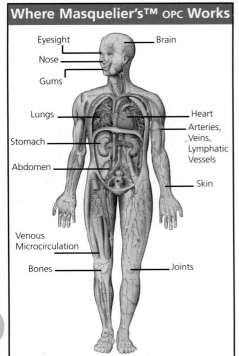

Where Masquelier's™ OPC Works

- Eyesight
- Nose
- Gums
- Brain
- Lungs
- Stomach
- Abdomen
- Heart
- Arteries, Veins, Lymphatic Vessels
- Skin
- Venous Microcirculation
- Bones
- Joints

compounds stimulate collagen and elastin production by cells, which reduces inflammation and can be beneficial in the treatment of arthritis and asthma.

In Europe, anthocyanins from bilberries are routinely prescribed by doctors before operations to prevent excessive post-operative bleeding (by up to 71 percent, according to German studies). Improved circulation brings enhanced mental clarity as well.

It is well-recognized that cranberry and blueberry anthocyanins are the most effective treatment and prevention for bladder and urinary tract infections; they can eliminate the need for using antibiotics to treat these conditions (although only under a physician's supervision).

Flavonoid-containing plants have been used for centuries to combat a wide range of conditions; clinical trials have now backed up this traditional knowledge. OPC flavonoids are active throughout your body, especially the heart, brain, lungs, arteries, veins, legs, capillaries, eyes, stomach, nose, bladder and urinary tract, gums, bones, lymphatic vessels, skin, and joints. We will look most closely at the heart and circulatory system. Flavonoids can help to protect your entire body from the ravages of the modern modern world and put a little colour into your life!

The Colour of the Cure . . . .

Most people in France know about OPCs and anthocyanins as top nutrients for treating varicose veins. They are also recognized as the active ingredients in grapes that make red wine so heart-healthy. Studies show that these flavonoids can actually strengthen veins and restore their elasticity–this makes varicose veins retract back into position. A scientific review published in 1995 by Italian researchers, plus over nine clinical trials have confirmed the efficacy of OPCs for treating varicose veins. One double-blind study of 50 patients with varicose veins showed that 150 mg of grape seed OPC daily worked faster and lasted longer than a commonly prescribed pharmaceutical drug (Diosmine) in reducing pain, sensations of burning and tingling, and the degree of distention of veins. All symptoms improved within 30 days. Myriad studies have also shown OPCs to reduce edema and swelling, which may be beneficial for persons suffering from high blood pressure, congestive heart failure, and sports injuries. OPCs have also been shown to be beneficial for treating eye strain, night blindness, macular degeneration, cancer, arthritis, asthma, spider veins, hay fever, allergies, nosebleeds, and gum disease.

The Role of Natural Medicine . . . .

The subject of heart health is very personal to me. When I was a young child, I lost both my parents within six years to preventable heart disease. In my mother's case, she was prescribed synthetic drugs. The side-effects from the treatment were so severe that she had to stop taking her medication. We now know that, in most cases, heart disease is preventable and reversible with diet and lifestyle changes. I believe that if my parents had known about the natural foods and herbs that can lower high blood pressure and strengthen the heart, my family's tragedy could have been avoided. Unfortunately, my experience with this disease is not rare. Heart disease, though largely preventable, is the leading cause of mortality in North America. This has been my inspiration to work countless hours to educate people about natural medicines.

The bilberry is the star performer when it comes to flavonoids that prevent heart disease.

9

What Are Flavonoids? . . . .

Over 6,000 different flavonoids have been identified in plants. All are powerful antioxidants because they contain polyphenol rings that can absorb free radicals, but some flavonoids have many other health benefits. Bioflavonoids, flavonoids with recognized biological activity, including rutin, hesperidin, and quercetin, are already considered essential for the processing of vitamin C within the body, the maintenance of capillary walls, and the fortification of collagen, the intercellular "cement" of the body. For instance, it is scientifically accepted that a deficiency of hesperidin in the diet is linked with abnormal capillary leakiness as well as pain in the extremities causing aches, weakness, and night leg-cramps.

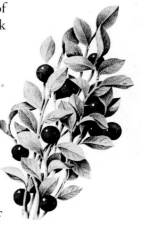

Randomized, double-blind, placebo-controlled clinical studies on each of these flavonoids have shown significant improvements for treating signs and symptoms of chronic venous insufficiency and cardiovascular disease. Treatment with rutin for two weeks also improved body temperature in one human study and was effective in controlling chronic venous hypertension, without side effects. Rutin can also: prevent the progression of micro-angiopathy to clinical stages; prevent neuropathy; treat hemorrhoids, and reduce plasma free radicals both locally and systemically. However, other important flavonoids, as discussed in this book, are just now beginning to be properly recognized.

What Are OPCs?

Let's look a bit more closely at these active ingredients concentrated in grapes, berries, and pine bark and how they work. In certain plants, a specific molecule (flavan-3-ol) bonds together to form entirely new molecules called oligomeric proanthocyanidins. By themselves, flavan-3-ol monomers (single units) can't be readily used by your body except as antioxidants. However, bonded together as oligomers (many units), these molecules become extremely biologically active and effective in the human body and provide a stunning array of health benefits.

Antioxidants and Free Radicals

Free radicals are highly reactive molecules capable of causing dramatic changes in the body, including cellular structural damage and the mutation and destruction of genetic material. The damage done by free radicals is irreversible. Free radicals are increased by injury, stress, pollution, and illness. The more free radicals are formed, the more antioxidants are needed to neutralize them. Nutritional antioxidants are free-radical scavengers or neutralizers that also prevent the formation of free radicals in the first place. A healthy body will produce healthy cells-and a balanced diet rich in antioxidants is the best form of protection against free-radical damage.

How Do Flavonoids Work in the Body?

Flavonoids (anthocyanins and OPCs) reduce blood platelet stickiness, prevent and reverse free-radical damage, improve the absorption of vitamin C by the body, and have a vitamin C sparing effect on the body. They also increase the body's production of collagen, elastin, and other compounds that form the basis of healthy blood vessel walls, skin, and connective tissues. Grape seed extract flavonoids and bilberry flavonoids can act to quickly repair and regenerate broken and leaky capillaries and blood vessels within the body.

Collagen lines the walls of our cardiovascular system and exists throughout the body in tissue membranes in the form of pairs of intertwined proteins and polypeptides. Collagen stability is determined by the cross-links that connect the intertwined strands.

Cross-linking is minimal in childhood (making skin soft) and increases as we grow older, in large part as a result of free-radical damage. Because flavonoids enhance the benefits of vitamin C, they stimulate the production of collagen in your body and enhance its recovery. Sixty percent of the protein found in the human body is collagen, so anything that helps with collagen structure and function can significantly improve health. Good collagen structure could be critical for preventing strokes.

Grape Flavonoids – Natural Blood Thinners

Heart attacks occur when blood clots stick to fatty deposits on the walls of the heart's arteries, choking off the supply of blood–so anything that can help to prevent blood platelet stickiness is desirable. While grapefruit and orange juice also contain plenty of flavonoids, they are different from the ones in purple grape juice.

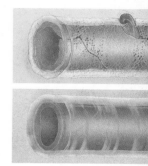

Every cell of the body has what is called a phospholipid membrane. Bilberry anthocyanins and grape seed OPCs quickly strengthen the walls of small vessels by forming complexes with these phospholipids.

11

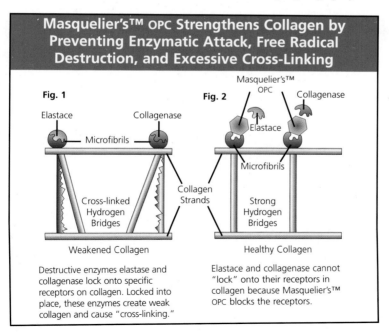

Masquelier's™ OPC Strengthens Collagen by Preventing Enzymatic Attack, Free Radical Destruction, and Excessive Cross-Linking

Fig. 1

Elastace — Collagenase
— Microfibrils —
Cross-linked Hydrogen Bridges
Collagen Strands
Weakened Collagen

Fig. 2

Masquelier's™ OPC — Collagenase
Elastace
— Microfibrils —
Strong Hydrogen Bridges
Healthy Collagen

Destructive enzymes elastase and collagenase lock onto specific receptors on collagen. Locked into place, these enzymes create weak collagen and cause "cross-linking."

Elastace and collagenase cannot "lock" onto their receptors in collagen because Masquelier's™ OPC blocks the receptors.

Researchers have compared grape with orange and grapefruit juice and came to the conclusion that grape juice is better for the heart. Clinical research with humans has shown that both ASA and red wine slow the activity of blood platelets by about 45 percent, while 9-12 oz of purple grape juice dampens them by about 75 percent. The anti-clotting effect of grape juice, also observed with OPC grape seed extract, pine bark extract, bilberry extract, cranberry and ginkgo, is due to specific flavonoids that inhibit blood platelet stickiness. And, unlike ASA, these compounds *do not increase bleeding time* and they actually help to prevent ulcers and gastrointestinal hemorrhage. Additionally, when people drink purple grape juice once a day, the benefits linger for several days so these flavonoids provide around-the-clock protection. Other studies have shown that Pycnogenol® pine bark extract inhibits platelet aggregation in a dose-dependent manner in humans, and the effect lasts for more than six days without increased bleeding time. Pycnogenol® also counteracts the constriction of blood vessels due to stress. The vaso-relaxant activity of Pycnogenol® is mediated through nitric oxide. Why not get a jump on these findings? Include flavonoid-rich foods in a healthy diet, which includes five to seven servings a day of vegetables, fruits, and juices. OPC supplements provide the myriad benefits of grapes and pine bark without all the sugar of grape juice or the alcohol of red wine. Consult a physician before stopping any medications as an extra added ounce of powerful prevention.

Flavonoids in Berries and Grapes

In the bilberry, five "parent" anthocyanins are found. Delphinidin is the predominant one; it has specific activity for eyesight as well as being a powerful antioxidant and having an affinity for collagen and elastin, improving circulatory problems. The anthocyanin profile of blueberry is very similar to that of bilberry, but has a lower concentration of anthocyanins because the anthocyanins are found only in the skin of the fruit; in bilberries anthocyanins are found throughout the pulp as well. Cranberry is characterized by a different anthocyanin profile and has the greatest effect on preventing bladder infections. Blueberry anthocyanins also can improve eyesight and relieve bladder infections but, of course, there is variation among blueberry species and cultivars. Grape skins have yet another anthocyanin profile.

All of these berries also contain pro-anthocyanidins, which are related to anthocyanins but have a neutral colour. Grape seeds and pine bark contain high levels of proanthocyanidins, which are powerful antioxidants and have therapeutic benefits similar to those of the anthocyanins.

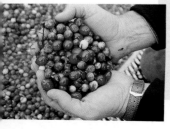

The flavonoids in cranberries have a great effect on preventing bladder infections.

Hawthorn for Heart Power

Our ancestors knew well the value of hawthorn leaves, flowers, and fruit for treating heart disease. Hawthorn (*Crataegus spp.*) is a member of the Rosaceae plant family, which includes apple, peach, almond, and strawberry. The "haws" from hawthorn trees and bushes, of which there are hundreds of species and varieties, are actually very similar to rosehips or tiny apples.

Hawthorn, which is also known as the mayflower, has been used as a folk medicine for the heart since the 14th century. Its list of uses includes treatment of congestive heart failure, atherosclerosis (plaque in the arteries), hypertension, and angina. Tonics from this plant can dilate coronary arteries, thus improving the heart's blood supply. One clinical trial based on a daily intake of 600 mg of hawthorn/passionflower extract (leaves, flowers, and fruits) corresponding to approximately three grams of the extract showed significant positive effects in a study with 78 patients with stage II heart failure.

Another clinical study with 132 stage II heart failure patients comparing hawthorn extract (900 mg per day) to an adequate low dosage of the conventional heart drug captopril showed no significant differences between the hawthorn treatment and the conventional drug using a rigorously controlled, multicentred and double-blind experimental design.

In another study of hawthorn, exercise capacity and improvements were evaluated. Significant improvements in exercise capacity were seen along with improvements in several physical parameters, including reduced total cholesterol levels and reduced breathlessness.

In Europe, hawthorn extracts are now being standardized for proanthocyanidin content. One delicious-tasting liquid hawthorn tonic produced by *Flora*, called Hawthorn Formula, contains a minimum of 30 mg of proanthocyanidins per daily dosage in a form that your body can use easily.

Both clinical studies and folk medicine support hawthorn as an effective heart medicine.

13

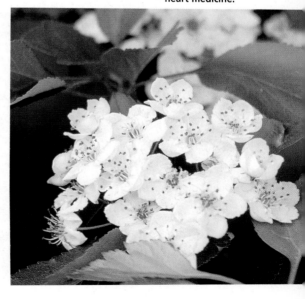

Flax Seed for Heart Health

Some heart-friendly seeds contain not flavonoids, but other substances that can improve the health of your cardiovascular system. Agriculture Canada, together with several Canadian medical researchers, has discovered that the seed coat of flax seed (*Linum usitatissimum*) contains a very beneficial plant estrogen called the SDG flax lignan, which quickly lowers cholesterol and reverses atherosclerosis (plaque in the arteries) caused by high cholesterol levels.

Several human trials have shown that flax seed lowers blood cholesterol in normal subjects and in those with high cholesterol. One controlled clinical trial with high-cholesterol subjects compared those who ate muffins containing 50 grams of defatted flax seed with subjects who ate muffins without flax seed (four muffins per day for *only three weeks*). The study found that flax seed has significant cholesterol-lowering effects: blood levels of LDL cholesterol (the bad kind) declined 9.3 percent in three weeks with flax.

Other studies on the flax lignan have shown that it can reduce total cholesterol, increase HDL cholesterol (the good one), reduce atherosclerosis due to high cholesterol, reduce diabetes mellitus, reduce endotoxic shock, and prevent the progression of lupus nephritis.

Flax seed oil is rich in omega-3 essential fatty acids. One study of 44 patients done in the 1980s on omega-3 deficiency found that flax had wide-ranging benefits for the cardiovascular system. The symptoms of two patients who had angina were completely relieved within several months. Three patients with high blood pressure reported decreases in their reading, and one patient with abnormally low blood pressure had her reading returned to normal while using flax seed oil. Another patient found relief of a severe varicose vein by applying flax seed oil directly to her leg.

Flax seed oil's omega-3 essential fatty acids can help bring balance to your essential fatty acid regulatory system, and it is that balance that is critical to health. Many people's diets contain too much omega-6 oil. Increasing your intake of omega-3 oils can correct that imbalance and protect you from heart disease. Both are essential, but they must be in balance.

A 1994 study reported in *The Lancet* found that a diet rich in alpha-linolenic acid, an omega-3 oil, reduced deaths from cardiovascular disease by an amazing 70 percent over a two-year period. Not bad for the humble flax seed! One thing to keep in mind when taking a flax seed oil supplement is that it is important to take a selenium supplement as well. Selenium is an omega-3 cofactor – you need it for the omega-3s to do their work properly and not cause further imbalance. For complete, easy-to-read information on this topic read *Fantastic Flax* by Siegfried Gursche (*alive* Health Guide #1, 2000).

Several studies have shown that flax seed lowers cholesterol.

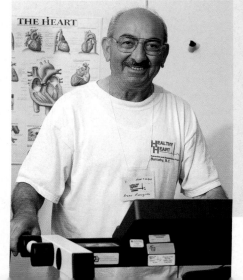

The Discovery of Flavonoids . . . .

Pine Bark Saves Cartier Expedition

Pine bark is a circulatory system healer that has been used for centuries. In one famous case, pine bark tea is reported to have saved the lives of the crewmen on Jacques Cartier's 1534 to 1535 expedition to present day Quebec. At the time, there was no medical understanding of the causes of scurvy, a disease that often afflicted sailors on long journeys when expedition provisions were limited to salted meat and dry biscuits. No fresh fruits or vegetables were available.

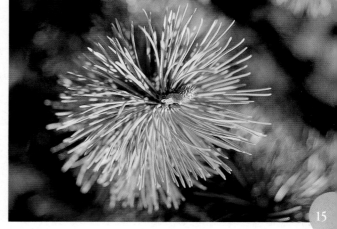

Ice-bound, with diminishing provisions, nearly all 110 men of Cartier's crew suffered from scurvy and twenty-five had already died. Scurvy's symptoms are a result of the body's inability to produce collagen. The first symptoms are fatigue, bleeding gums, and loose teeth. Eventually, tissues begin to hemorrhage. If left untreated, scurvy is usually fatal within six months. The direct cause of death is usually gangrene, caused by poor circulation.

Pine bark has been used as a circulatory system healer for centuries.

Cartier's expedition was saved thanks to the medicinal knowledge of the Iroquoians of a nearby village. The Iroquoians recognized the crew's symptoms and taught Cartier how to prepare an extract and poultice from the needles and bark of the "anneda" tree.

Cartier experimented with this remedy on two men, who recovered within a week. The rest of the expedition was given the same remedy, and survived.

In Search of Vitamin C and...Vitamin P?

Albert Szent-Györgyi (1893-1986), Hungarian-born American biochemist, molecular biologist, and Nobel Prize winner, is known for many contributions during his long and varied scientific career. Szent-Györgyi was awarded the 1937 Nobel Prize in medicine for demonstrating how cells obtain energy and for his work in isolating vitamin C. But Szent-Györgyi was well aware that the whole secret hadn't been unraveled yet and that, in terms of healing scurvy, the name vitamin C lent too much credit to ascorbic acid for curing the disease.

So he continued his search for the mysterious anti-scurvy cofactor. In 1936, he and his colleagues managed to extract a complex substance from the peels of lemons. They called it "citrin." Citrin contained vitamin C and a mixture of other compounds, which Szent-Györgyi was unable to isolate and identify.

Experiments were conducted with citrin, and it was discovered that it possessed vascular wall-strengthening properties. The collapse of vascular walls is one of the main problems in scurvy. Because citrin did a much better job than vitamin C at fixing this problem, Szent-Györgyi decided he had found a new vitamin. He took the "P" from the word "permeability" and baptized the extract vitamin P. However, citrin never acquired true vitamin status because later experiments failed to demonstrate a condition of citrin deficiency.

During the rest of his life, Szent-Györgyi never refuted the idea that scurvy may be caused by a lack of vitamin C plus a cofactor. Szent-Györgyi is quoted as saying that the unknown vitamin P found in the pine bark given to Jacques Cartier's men was more powerful and more important than vitamin C for preventing the permeability of blood vessels and ultimately reversing the effects of scurvy. When shown the research on proanthocyanidins done by Professor Jacques Masquelier of France, Szent-Györgyi is said to have conceded that proanthocyanidins were the elusive vitamin P compounds he had looked for in pine bark.

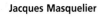

Jacques Masquelier

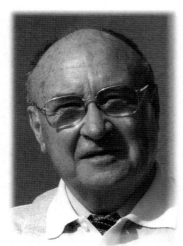

The Discovery of Proanthocyanidins in Peanut Skins

In the mid-1940s, Jacques Masquelier was beginning his medical studies at the Bordeaux Medical University in France. As a part of his PhD work, he was asked to determine whether or not it was safe

16

to feed cattle the papery skins found on peanuts.

During the war, peanut skins were a common waste product of the peanut oil-pressing industry, and there was interest in recycling these by-products instead of just throwing them away. Masquelier received samples of the peanut skins and found that they were a concentrated source of bitter-tasting, more or less colourless flavonoids. He first called these flavonoids leukoanthocyanidins, literally meaning "pale anthocyanins" ("leuko" means "pale" in Latin).

To determine if these compounds were safe to eat, he did studies with guinea pigs, and it was then that he discovered their remarkable capillary-strengthening effects. To study this, Masquelier did what I like to call "the hickey test;" he fed the guinea pigs the concentrated peanut skin extract and then exposed a small area of skin to suction.

He had determined that capillaries normally burst at a certain suction pressure resulting in the formation of a characteristic red patch of skin, or "hickey." But when he had given the guinea pigs the concentrated leukoanthocyanidin extract, he had to apply much more pressure before the capillaries burst. Capillary strength was seen to double even within hours of orally giving the extract!

It was soon clear from these and other studies that the peanut skins were indeed safe and that, far from being toxic, even at high dosages, the concentrated leukoanthocyanidin extracts that Masquelier and his colleagues had isolated had dramatic circulatory-strengthening effects. It so happened that at the time of these studies, the wife of Masquelier's professor was pregnant and was suffering from terrible edema (swelling often due to water retention) of her ankles and knees, a condition frequently suffered by pregnant women.

Masquelier and his PhD supervisor knew that edema is caused by broken and leaky blood vessels and capillaries, and so they decided to see how well their extracts worked for the woman's painful and debilitating condition (she could barely walk). Much to their delight, she was completely cured within 48 hours! And so it was, in the early 1950s in France, that the first standardized leukoanthocyanidin (OPC) product, called Resivit, was created from peanut skin extract and put on the market for treating circulatory disorders. This product is still available today.

Peanut skins are a concentrated source of colourless flavonoids called leukoanthocyanidins (literally translated as pale anthocyanidins), later renamed proanthocyanidins.

After Masquelier discovered OPCs in 1947, he went on to look for other sources and found that these flavonoids are everywhere in the plant kingdom; they are especially concentrated in grape seeds, grape skins, grape leaves, and pine bark. Masquelier also discovered that often when leaves turn red in the fall, it is because of an enzymatic reaction that happens when the weather becomes cooler, changing OPCs (colourless) into red anthocyanins. This chemical reaction, which can be re-created in the laboratory, has become the definitive test for detecting the presence of these flavonoids in different plant materials.

Studies done by Masquelier confirmed that OPCs can extend lifespan tremendously even in starvation situations, let alone during times of mere vitamin C deficiency. Perhaps this explains why animals such as deer and moose can often survive in extreme winter conditions for months on end just by eating tree bark, which is a rich source of proanthocyanidins. Elephants and giraffes, even though they are large and tall, have excellent circulation and cardiovascular health when they live in the wild and eat their natural diet of tree bark and leaves.

Tea, Cocoa, Almonds, and Nuts Good for Heart Health

Tea drinkers can be happy to know that they are benefiting from flavonoids with every delicious cup! Although tea doesn't contain OPCs it does provide some heart-health benefits. Based on clinical research, drinking five cups of black tea daily for three weeks can reduce total cholesterol by up to 7 percent and LDL cholesterol by up to 11 percent compared with a placebo drink (with or without caffeine). According to researchers, this could translate into an 8 percent to 13 percent decreased risk of heart disease. However, tea did not affect the patients' antioxidant levels.

Grandmas will be pleased to learn that for every cup of hot cocoa they prepare they are serving up generous heart-health benefits. Cocoa flavonoids inhibit low-density lipoprotein oxidation, reduce thrombosis (blood clots), improve vascular function, and reduce inflammation. Chemical analysis has shown that

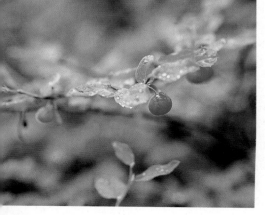

Anthocyanins and OPCs are found in huckleberries.

18

cocoa has the highest levels of antioxidants per serving (564 mg of flavonoids), twice as high as red wine (163 mg of flavonoids), and nearly three times stronger than green tea (47 mg of flavonoids) or black tea (34 mg of flavonoids). A cup of hot cocoa is low in saturated fats (0.3 g per serving) compared with a chocolate bar (8 g per 40 g bar), and the heat may help trigger release of more antioxidants.

Nut lovers will also be glad to hear that a daily handful of yummy almonds also benefits the cardiovascular system. Based on clinical studies, about one handful of almonds daily decreases LDL "bad" cholesterol by 4.4 percent while with two handfuls of almonds–accounting for a little less than a quarter of the day's total calories–LDL cholesterol drops by 9.4 percent. According to experts, that may reduce the risk of heart disease in the long run by 30 percent. Nuts contain high levels of heart-healthy unsaturated fats that are known to lower LDL cholesterol levels in the blood and reduce the risk of heart disease. Nuts also contain phytosterols (plant sterols) such as beta sitosterol that lower cholesterol.

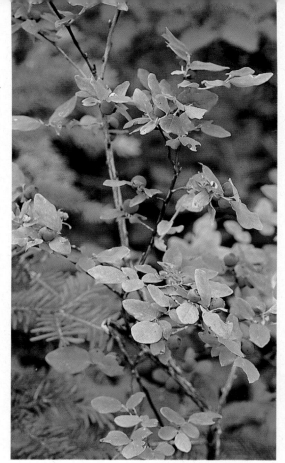

Wild blueberries, such as the oval-leaved blueberry, are the most concentrated common food sources of flavonoids.

Bilberry and wild blueberries are the most concentrated common food sources of flavonoids, with red wine and green tea following (with less than half the amounts). Dried bilberries contain approximately 0.7 percent anthocyanins.

Research looking at several of the wild blueberry and bilberry species of the coastal old-growth forests of British Columbia has determined that dried Alaskan blueberries contain as much as 3.4 percent anthocyanins, mountain bilberries contain 2.8 percent, and oval-leaved blueberries contain 2.2 percent. Commercial blueberries generally have only 0.2 percent anthocyanins.

Pycnogenol®

Pycnogenol® is the extract of the bark of the Maritime pine, which grows in southern France. This product is a compound of forty substances, including proanthocyanidins.

Several placebo-controlled human studies have shown that Pycnogenol® pine bark extract can quickly improve circulation and prevent leg and ankle edema and blood clots caused by long airplane flights. Most people will notice the effects of in-flight swelling if they take their shoes off during a flight and have difficulty getting back into them at the end of the flight. This effect of flying is well known-and it can also increase the risk of potentially deadly blood clots, strokes, and embolisms. Simply taking 200mg of Pycnogenol® two hours before flights, another 200mg six hours later, and 100mg the next day was able to prevent this problem by strengthening veinous walls. Pycnogenol enables veins that are stretched by pooled blood to better resist increased pressure, letting less liquid seep into tissues and reducing swelling and edema.

Pycnogenol®, a patented product, works its magic by inhibiting adrenaline-induced blood platelet aggregation (clumping and clotting) and by shielding the lining of arteries against injury. These effects are what lower blood pressure and protect against heart disease. It also increases circulation and therefore inhibits inflammation. And if inflammation is already present, it can reduce it, thus treating varicose veins.

Here's one woman's story: This patient suffered from an irregular heart beat, elevated blood pressure, and chronic fatigue syndrome (which is thought to be related to an abnormality of blood pressure regulation and free-radical damage to the adrenal glands). After just six weeks of using Pycnogenol®, her heart beat and blood pressure symptoms had improved by a dramatic 80 percent.

Grape seed OPCs are closely related to Pycnogenol® (pine bark extract). These compounds remain in the blood stream for up to three days and patrol your system and protect the body from damage by quenching free radicals incorporated into your tissues and cells. They also aid the repair system of the body.

Grape & Berry Flavonoid Products and Dosages

One thing that Masquelier stressed is that not all grape seed extracts are the same. The extract he developed, called OPC-85™, is a 98-percent pure antioxidant complex made up of different types of proanthocyanidins with a specific breakdown of each.

According to Masquelier's research, all proanthocyanidins are powerful antioxidants, but it is only the OPCs that are active in the repair of collagen and the strengthening of blood vessels and capillaries. They also have the strongest antibacterial and antiviral properties (preventing bacteria from sticking to cell membranes and viruses from penetrating into cells) and can prevent histamine

How Free Radicals Disrupt Normal Cellular Functions

Free radicals breaking lysosomal membrane. Histamine leaks out.

Free radicals breaking nuclear membrane altering DNA (genetic) material.

Free radicals attacking cell membrane from inside. Easy entry for destructive enzymes and pollutants

release through protection of immune cells against degradation by enzymes (important for alleviating allergies and hayfever). To obtain the full cardiovascular and other benefits reported here, it is imperative that you use a well-researched extract standardized for OPC content.

Similarly, studies with the colourful flavonoids (anthocyanins) from bilberries showed a 50 percent strengthening of capillaries within only four hours in studies done with rats!

Another study looked at the effects of bilberry extract (standardized to contain 25 percent anthocyanins) on reducing blood platelet aggregation.

Masquelier's® OPC-85™ Grape Seed Extract The recommended dosage for Masquelier's® OPC-85™ Grape Seed Extract is 300 mg daily for ten to fourteen days (especially for people suffering from serious coronary artery disease and allergies), then 100 mg daily thereafter. In studies reporting significant results, long-term daily dosages range from 100 mg (for treating venous-lymphatic insufficiency) to 300 mg (for eye strain from staring at a computer screen).

Masquelier's® OPC-85™ Grape Seed Extract was tested double-blind on a group of elderly people with fragile capillaries, and 79 percent had significant improvement after two weeks with only 100 to 150 mg per day.

Clinical studies on humans indicate that 300 mg per day of OPC-85™ can quickly repair broken, leaky blood vessels and thus alleviate water retention and edema (puffy eyes, swollen feet, bloating associated with premenstrual syndrome, etc).

Flavonoid Heart Medicine: What to Take		
Condition	**Product**	**Dosage**
Cardiovascular disease	Pycnogenol®	25 mg/25 lb body weight for 10 days then 100 mg/day
Coronary artery disease	OPC-85™	300 mg/day for 10-14 days
Fragile capillaries	OPC-85™	100-150 mg/day for 14 days
Leaky blood vessels	OPC-85™	300 mg/day
Platelet aggregation	25% bilberry extract	80-160 mg 3 times/day
Poor circulation	Pycnogenol®	25 mg/25 lb body weight for 10 days then 100 mg/day
Varicose veins	25% bilberry extract OR Pycnogenol®	500 mg/day OR 25 mg/25 lb body weight for 10 days then 100 mg/day
Venous-lymphatic insufficiency	OPC-85™	100 mg/day

As with all supplements, discuss taking flavonoids with your health-care provider before beginning any treatment. If you are taking medication, do not discontinue it without talking to your doctor.

The dosage was 80 to 160 mg three times daily. The researchers concluded that bilberry extract does in fact reduce platelet aggregation.

Other research showed that patients suffering from varicose veins and ulcerative dermatitis showed a substantial drop in capillary leakage after they took bilberry extract standardized to contain 25 percent anthocyanins; the dosage was 480 mg daily. Anthocyanins were found to protect capillary walls and to restore the altered sheath of the capillary.

Pycnogenol® is usually taken in a loading or saturation dose of 25 mg per 25 pounds of body weight for up to six weeks (usually seven to ten days), then reduced depending on the particular condition being treated.

OPC Products

OPC-85™ is the original grape seed extract researched by Dr. Masquelier. Each capsule of the product *Beyond Grape Seed (OPC-85™ Grape Seed Extract Plus Bilberry)* contains: 50 mg of OPC-85 grape seed extract (standardized to contain 98 percent proanthocyanidins and 65 percent OPCs); 10 mg of bilberry extract (standardized to 25 percent anthocyanins) in a base of 290 mg freeze-dried cranberry powder. Masquelier's® OPC extract has been manufactured since the 1970s at the same plant in France, so you are guaranteed a scientifically substantiated source of grape seed extract.

Bilberry Products

One excellent bilberry supplement is *Floravision*. Each capsule contains 250 mg of bilberry extract standardized to 25 percent anthocyanins in a whole-food base of freeze-dried blueberry powder. One capsule is guaranteed to provide a therapeutic dose of anthocyanins, unlike many other bilberry products and eyesight formulas on the market. There are a number of other products available that contain lower concentrations of anthocyanins that may not be therapeutic. Be sure the product you buy has not been sterilized with methyl bromide or treated with ethylene oxide. These widely used fumigants are known to leave carcinogenic residues on exposed foods and food supplements (*Flora* does not use this method on any of its products).

Each Floravision capsule provides a therapeutic dose of anthocyanins.

23

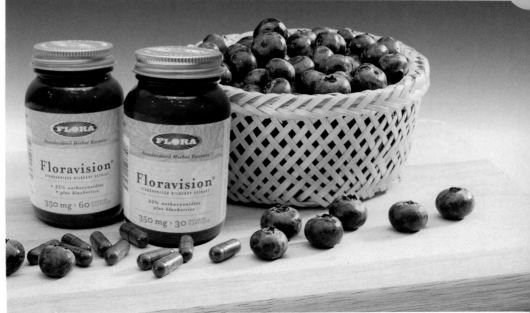

How Else Are Flavonoids Important to Health?

We've seen the benefits flavonoids can have for your heart and circulatory system, but these amazing substances can do much more for your body. In fact, the discovery and understanding of flavonoids could be the biggest medical breakthrough since the discovery of penicillin. Other therapeutic uses for anthocyanins and OPCs include the treatment of the following:

- Acne
- AIDS
- Alcoholism
- Allergies
- Alzheimer's disease
- Anxiety
- Athlete's foot
- Attention-deficit disorder
- Bed wetting
- Bladder infections
- Blood toxicity
- Cancer
- Diabetes
- Diarrhea
- Dysfunctional immune system
- High cholesterol
- Poor vision
- Premenstrual syndrome
- Signs of aging
- Stress

Recent findings have concluded that OPCs and berry flavonoids are the most powerful antioxidants available for the treatment and prevention of disease. According to one former cardiac surgeon, "There is no reason why you can't live to 120!"

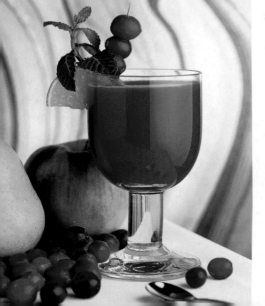

Canadian nurse Phyllis I. Dales, RN, NUA, author of the book *Cranberry: The Cure for Common and Chronic Conditions*, knows well the power of cranberry flavonoids to help cure recurrent kidney and bladder infections. Phyllis had chronic UTIs (Urinary Tract Infections) and had tried a myriad of different antibiotics but nothing worked until she tried cranberry. Even her medical doctor admits that she would likely be on kidney dialysis without cranberry. She believes cranberries saved her life.

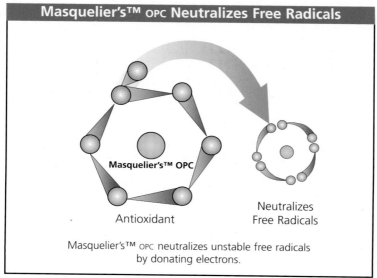

Masquelier's™ OPC Neutralizes Free Radicals

Masquelier's™ OPC

Antioxidant

Neutralizes
Free Radicals

Masquelier's™ OPC neutralizes unstable free radicals
by donating electrons.

Antioxidant Properties

OPCs are powerful antioxidants that help prevent oxidative damage to cellular membranes. They help to protect cellular and tissue membranes from free radical-initiated damage and possess free-radical scavenging capacity superior to that of other known antioxidants, such as vitamins C and E. OPCs are readily used by the body and can penetrate all types of cellular membranes to offer protection against cellular damage by all types of free radicals, and against free-radical initiated chemical reactions.

Aging Skin

OPCs support collagen production, a vital factor in maintaining healthy-looking skin. They protect against the breakdown of skin collagen, a process that produces visible signs of aging. They also help the body to preserve collagen protein and enhance the elasticity of skin. Their pro-circulatory function is active in the skin as well.

For Athletes

OPCs have special benefits for active people. They are essential to minimizing sports injury recovery times and they enhance the body's recovery following strenuous workouts.

Nature's Sun Screens

One of the functions of anthocyanins and OPCs in plants is to act as a screen against damaging ultraviolet radiation. There is evidence that anthocyanins and proanthocyanidins confer their sun-protective effects to the eyes and skin of those who ingest them. These powerful antioxidants reduce ultraviolet-B radiation damage in proportion to the amount of antioxidant present, so the more of them you eat, the better protected you are from the sun's damaging rays. Their primary activity is through their excellent capacity to capture superoxide radicals and stimulate protective enzymes in cells such as SOD. Anthocyanins form a protective barrier around cell membranes, which block destructive enzymes and free radicals that would otherwise cause cell damage.

Vision Problems

As we have seen, anthocyanins possess protective properties related to circulation. In addition to being critical to heart health, this is also particularly important to the health of the eye, the location of the highest density of the finest capillaries in the body.

The therapeutic value of certain blue anthocyanins for improving vision was discovered during World War II when Royal Air Force pilots noticed a definite advantage over the enemy on night flights after they consumed bilberry jam or pie. Clinical trials have verified this and revealed that the blue pigments in bilberry increase the pigment needed in the retina for night vision within an hour of eating these foods! No wonder RAF pilots were given a ration of these berries before night flights.

Since that time, further research has confirmed that bilberry anthocyanins are powerful agents for improving eyesight, including night vision. Bilberries and standardized bilberry extracts are also effective for treating other eyesight disorders, which are often linked to poor circulation in the eye.

The blue pigments in bilberry increase the pigment needed in the retina for night vision.

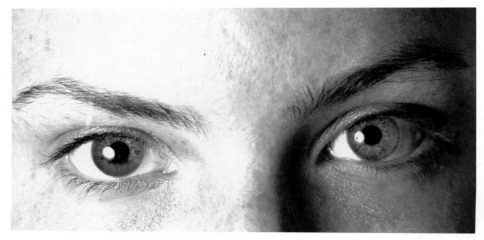

In one study, bilberry extract improved eyesight and increased blood supply to the eye in 75 percent of patients. It has been shown to improve nearsightedness after five months of regular use, while an 83 percent improvement in visual acuity was recorded after only 15 days. Bilberry extract also has the ability to stop cataracts: in 48 out of 50 patients, treatment with bilberry extract and vitamin E arrested the progression of their age-related cortical cataracts. Long-term improvements took an average of six weeks with regular doses of a standardized 25 percent anthocyanin extract. Bilberry acts to improve vision through the same mechanisms that improve your heart health by

- improving capillary strength
- reducing capillary leakage
- thinning the blood by reducing platelet stickiness.

The resulting improved blood flow is essential for optimum vision.

Treatment of Eye Conditions

Bilberry anthocyanins are recommended at a dosage of between 200 and 800 mg per day for various problems. One study using a single oral dose of 200 mg of bilberry extract in 22 patients suffering from myopia, glaucoma, or retinitis pigmentosa showed that the subjects had improvements, based on the results of electroretinography (a method of checking activity in the retina).

Bilberries and standardized bilberry extracts are effective for treating eyesight disorders.

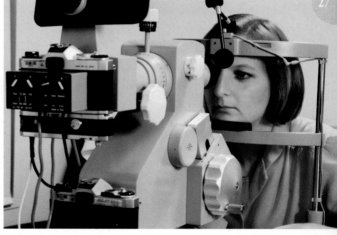

The results of those patients with retinitis pigmentosa, however, were inconclusive in this limited study. Other researchers studied the effects of 400 mg per day of bilberry anthocyanins, together with 20 mg per day of betacarotene, on 33 patients suffering from vision disorders, including 11 with retinitis pigmentosa, and they demonstrated improved adaptation to light and night vision and enlargement of the visual field.

Another excellent product for improving eyesight is Vision Factors by Natural Factors that combines BlueRichTM blueberry extract, bilberry extract, grapeseed extract, lutein, zeaxanthin, zinc, vitamin C, and other important vitamins and minerals critical for proper eye health. All nutrients are present in a therapeutic dosage range including 7.5mg per capsule of natural lutein from marigold flowers (Tagetes erecta). Lutein and its companion carotenoid, zeaxanthin, are the only carotenoids found in the human lens, and these colorful antioxidants are critical for preventing cataracts. Their role is also central in preventing oxidative damage to the area of the retina responsible for fine vision. Supplementing the diet with 10 to 15 mg of lutein daily can improve visual function including glare recovery, contrast sensitivity, and visual acuity versus placebo and may also prevent glaucoma.

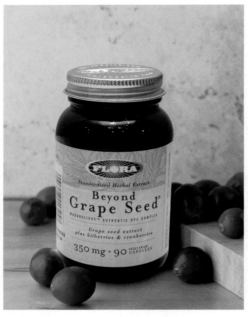

The anthocyanins in certain berries, especially cranberries, prevent bladder problems.

Bladder Infections

Bilberry, blueberry, and cranberry anthocyanins prevent bladder problems and are proven to be effective in the treatment of urinary tract infections. The anthocyanins in these berries prevent bacteria from adhering to the lining of the bladder and urinary tract. The effective dose for treating urinary tract infections is just two glasses of 25 percent real fruit juice per day. This simple addition to your diet will also help provide the myriad other positive benefits of anthocyanins.

Diarrhea

Bilberries and blueberries can easily be used to combat diarrhea with their powerful antibiotic activity. The bacteria they fight include *E. coli*, a common cause of diarrhea. In Europe, blueberry soup made with a third of an ounce of berries is a traditional cure for diarrhea. Powdered bilberry can also be used effectively for treating dyspepsia (stomach problems) in infants. Again, these antibiotic effects are most likely due to the ability of these flavonoids to prevent bacteria from sticking to cell walls.

Diabetes

Diabetics have long known of the many benefits of bilberry for improving circulation. Studies have documented bilberry's efficacy for reducing thickenings of capillaries due to abnormal collagen and glycoprotein production, a condition characteristic of diabetes. In one study, 54 patients were given 50 to 600 mg per day of the berry extract for between eight and 33 months. This treatment produced an almost total normalization of these conditions.

A specific proanthocyanidin called myrtillin, which is found in bilberry leaf, significantly reduces hyperglycemia and can normalize blood sugar levels in some diabetics. Bilberry leaf tea was one of the top treatments for diabetes before the discovery of insulin. Although less potent than insulin, it is considered by some researchers to be less damaging to the body than insulin with long-term use. The recommended dosage of myrtillin is one gram per day. A single dose can produce blood sugar balancing effects lasting for several weeks (Diabetics should *not* stop taking their insulin while trying this).

One doctor reviewed the treatment of 60 diabetic patients. In 36 cases the myrtillin was believed to be beneficial, because it was possible to make the patients' diets less restrictive, decrease their insulin, or both.

Isoflavonoids from Beans and Legumes

Isoflavonoids such as genistein from soy, red clover, and kudzu root are called phytoestrogens (plant estrogens). These beneficial flavonoids not only have dramatic anticancer effects, they also lower cholesterol, help to reverse atherosclerosis, improve calcium metabolism, reduce cravings, and prevent many other diseases. Isoflavonoids have been shown to safely support "estrogen homeostasis" in both men and women, which is important for calcium metabolism and is fundamental to tissue health throughout the body. Extensive controlled clinical trials have documented dramatic anticancer effects for a synthetic drug called phenoxodiol which is

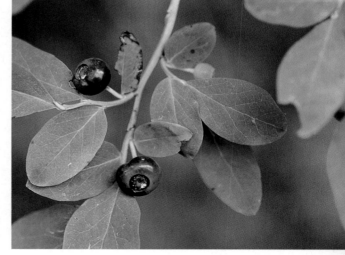

Bilberries and blueberries, such as the Alaskan blueberry, contain powerful antibiotic activity.

29

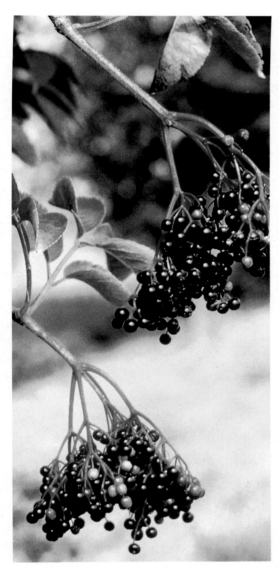

Elderberry is a proven remedy for combating the common flu virus.

based on a red clover isoflavonoid metabolite naturally produced when certain isoflavones are consumed. Phenoxodiol is active against most major forms of human cancer so far tested, including prostate cancer (strong anti-cancer effects have also been documented with Promensil natural red clover extract). Red clover isoflavonoids also have proven clinical efficacy for treating high cholestrerol, cardiovascular disease, osteoporosis, endometriosis, fibroids, hot flashes, menopausal problems, and other hormone-related diseases. Soy isoflavonoid extracts have been shown in human clinical trials to be comparable to some diabetes drugs. They not only lower blood sugar but also lower cholesterol. Berries and grape products also contain beneficial phytoestrogens including the compound, resveratrol. Part of why phytoestrogens are active against cancer and so many other diseases may come down to a calcium-estrogen connection. According to Dr. Takuo Fujita, MD, Calcium Research Institute, Institute of Science and Technology, Japan, calcium deficiency not only causes osteoporosis, but also interferes with signal transduction of cells and estrogen activity and can cause increased intracellular calcium and diseases including high blood pressure, arteriosclerosis, diabetes mellitus, Alzheimer's disease, mood swings, PMS, kidney stones, and cancer. It is important to note that probiotic supplements should be taken in order to maximize the benefits of phytoestrogens.

Colds and Flu

We've talked mostly about the flavonoids found in grape seed extract, bilberries, and pine bark, but there are other great sources of these flavonoids. One of these is elderberry, which can treat a number of conditions. Traditionally, elderberry has been used to treat colds, coughs, and upper respiratory tract infections, but the lectins and anthocyanins present in elderberry also help protect cells from free-radical damage, slowing down the aging process and strengthening the immune system.

Recent clinical studies proved that elderberry was effective in combating the common flu virus and have shown that the anthocyanins from elderberries actually prevent viral particles from getting into cells and multiplying.

Lifestyle Choices: Heart-Healthy Tips . . . .

While taking flavonoids will greatly improve heart health, they do not replace the importance of healthful lifestyle choices. Diet, for example, and getting adequate daily vitamins and minerals preferably from natural sources is fundamental to heart health.

Avoid the simple carbohydrates found in foods that contain white flour and sugar. Instead, eat whole foods.

Blood Sugar and Insulin

The cardiovascular system is damaged by large swings in blood sugar and insulin. It is important to realize that insulin, although vital in normal amounts, is considered by medical researchers to be a deadly "aging bombshell" in excess. Avoid the simple carbohydrates found in white bread, white sugar, white pasta, and other highly processed foods (and the spikes and troughs of blood sugar and insulin they cause). Instead, eat the complex carbohydrates found in whole grains and minimally processed foods in order to maintain more gradual changes in blood sugar and insulin levels.

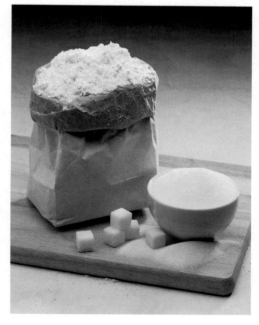

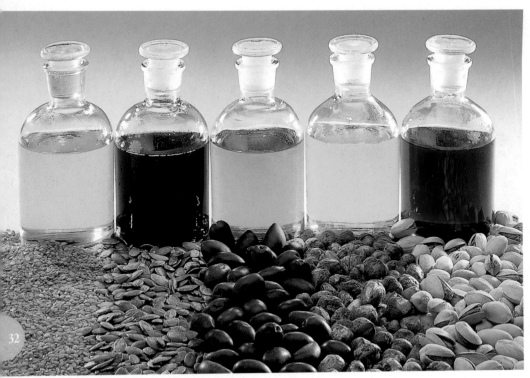

**Essential fatty acids are
absolutely *essential* for
good health.**

Essential Fatty Acids

There is much talk these days about the benefits of a low- or
no-fat diet, but, in fact, certain fats are absolutely essential for
good health. Few people appreciate just how important "good"
fats are for health, and conversely just how detrimental "bad"
fat–or not enough good fats–in the diet can be. Fat is not some-
thing that should be avoided. There are two fatty acids that are
essential for life: linoleic acid in the omega-6 oil family, and
alpha-linolenic acid in the omega-3 oil family.

Like vitamins, these essential fatty acids can't be produced by
the body and therefore must be obtained through the diet.
Linoleic acid is found in certain seed oils, while alpha-linolenic
acid is found mainly in dark green leafy vegetables and flax seed
oil. Linoleic acid and alpha-linolenic acid must be obtained from
foods in the proper balance because they are required for the production of many biologically essential molecules.

To be useful to the body, these two essential fatty acids must be converted by a series of steps in the body to other kinds of fatty acids. These conversions can be slowed down by many lifestyle factors, including a diet rich in saturated fats and trans fatty acids, stress, viral infections, too much alcohol or cholesterol, and various illnesses.

Together, linoleic acid and alpha-linolenic acid in an approximately equal ratio should comprise at least 5 percent of your daily calories (especially for children), but the average North American diet often does not provide this absolute requirement for health. It is estimated that most people are deficient in essential fatty acids, especially the omega-3 type, which protect the body against abnormal clotting and have anti-inflammatory properties.

Every cell of the body has a phospholipid membrane and that lipid layer is made up of essential fatty acids: 60 percent in most cells and 80 percent for brain and nerve cells. Studies have shown that increased levels of omega-3 oils in the diet increase the flexibility of red blood cells for passing through capillaries and blood vessels *within only three days* and reduce or normalize blood platelet stickiness. This translates into a 27 percent reduced risk of heart attack for those who are at high risk of an attack, while a low-fat or high-fiber diet has no effect on reducing risk of heart attack.

Incorporate flax oil, hemp seed oil, and fish into the diet. For complete, easy-to-understand information about essential fatty acids read *Good Fats and Oils*, by Siegfried Gursche (***alive*** Natural Health Guide #17, 2000).

Eat Celery to Reverse High Blood Pressure

Celery has been shown to lower blood pressure.

Did you know that celery has been used as a medicine for lowering blood pressure by Asian cultures since 200 BC? The active compound is what gives celery its aroma. It has been shown to lower blood pressure by 12 to 14 percent in a few weeks based on animal studies and lowers cholesterol levels by about 14 percent at the same time. One 62-year-old man ate two stalks of celery every day for a week and his blood pressure dropped from a high 158/96 to a normal 118/82.

Heart Disease Prevention is of number one interest in North America. And it should be! According to the Heart and Stroke Foundation, 32% of all male deaths in Canada in 2002 were due to heart diseases, diseases of the blood vessels, and stroke. For women, the toll was even higher: 34% of all female deaths in 2002 were due to cardiovascular disease. In 1999, 20,926 people died of heart attacks in Canada and 21,693 died of coronary disease. There were 13,215 deaths from congestive heart failure; and out of 50,000 stroke victims that year, 15,409 died. Every year there are between 70 to 120 heart bypass surgeries performed per 100,000 people across Canada. In the United States, the numbers are even more staggering. And while men were once statistically most at risk of heart disease the American Heart Association (AHA), now claims that nearly 500,000 women in the US die each year of heart complications! This is more than the next seven leading causes of death combined, including cancer!

The only remedy against heart disease and stroke is change of diet and lifestyle!

The latest recommendations from the AHA, endorsed by more than 30 other organizations, is to call for those whose health is a concern to themselves and their doctors to adopt a personal and preventive approach. Lifestyle factors known to reduce

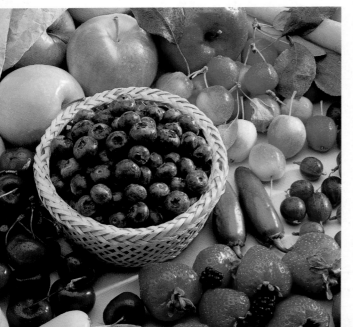

the risk of heart disease are vital: these are stopping smoking; regular exercise of at least 30 minutes several times per week; a heart-healthy diet that includes plenty of fruits, vegetables, and whole grains; limiting saturated fats; avoiding *trans* fats altogether; and maintaining a healthy weight. While AHA also recommends supplementing the diet with omega-3 fatty acids and folic acid for people at high risk, in addition to taking ASA and heart medications, the researchers erroneously recommend against antioxidants because of what they call "lack of proof!" They obviously know nothing about the latest flavonoid research being done by one of the world's leading heart specialists, Dr. John Folts of the US. Scientific study also backs the isoflavonoids from soy, red clover, kudzu root, and other legumes as well as the closely related lignans from flax seeds which naturally lower high cholesterol and reverse atherosclerosis while also providing strong anticancer, antidiabetic, and hormone-balancing effects. Heart health also depends on an adequate daily allowance of minerals and vitamins, especially magnesium and vitamin E.

It is never too late to begin. Many people have been able to avoid heart bypass surgery and achieve optimum health with daily use of antioxidants and other food-based therapies described in this book. American cardiac surgeon Dr. Robert Willix, MD. reports that he has exchanged his scalpel for prescribing antioxidants, and especially flavonoids, for prevention of heart disease and aging. He gave up heart surgery when he discovered one patient's arteries were too hard even to cut with the scalpel. He told the patient to go home, work in the garden, do other gentle exercise, and eat foods rich in flavonoids. That man recovered completely–and Dr. Willix went on to dramatically change his practice.

This book will show you how to vastly improve your own cardiovascular health and avoid heart surgery with flavonoid-rich foods and supplements. (The publishers recommend this approach for heart patients should only be taken under a physician's supervision.)

A personal note from the author: . . . .

Based on all of the research that I have seen, I think of grapes and berries like bilberries, blueberries, and strawberries as perhaps being God's idea of pills–delicious and nutritious and filled with a bountiful cornucopia of beneficial compounds that help us stay youthful, vital and healthy. It's time for people to wake up and for both doctors and the medical profession generally to educate themselves to the proven benefits of antioxidants and flavonoids for preventing heart disease. Governments must support further clinical research on flavonoids and other natural remedies for improving cardiovascular health.

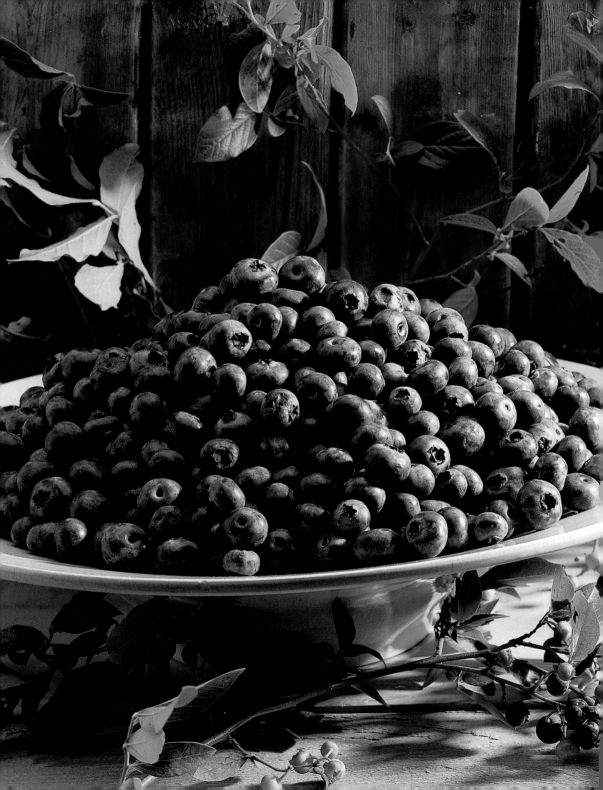

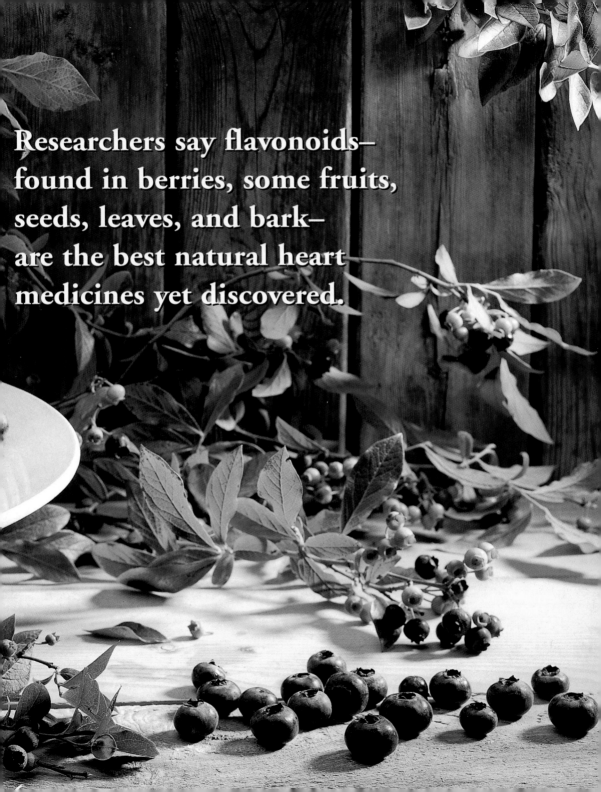

Researchers say flavonoids—
found in berries, some fruits,
seeds, leaves, and bark—
are the best natural heart
medicines yet discovered.

Mixed Berries
and Exotic Fruit with Yogurt

Served as breakfast, this "taste of the day" will energize your body and the fresh enjoyable taste will stay with you for a long time; as a snack after a hard day's work, it'll replenish the vitamins and minerals needed for a robust heart muscle. Berries are an excellent source of flavonoids, which help repair blood vessels, reduce blood platelet clotting, protect against free-radical damage and improve vitamin C absorption.

1 tsp (5 ml)
fresh lemon juice

1 Tbsp (15 ml) **honey**

2 cups (500 ml)
natural yogurt or kefir

½ **cup** (125 ml)
blueberries

½ **cup** (125 ml)
blackberries

½ **cup** (125 ml)
strawberries, quartered

½ **cup** (125 ml) **yellow
plum, quartered**

½ **cup** (125 ml) **lychees,
peeled**

2 Tbsp (15 ml) **sunflower
or pumpkin seeds,
toasted**

Fresh mint, for garnish

In a bowl, combine lemon and honey then stir in yogurt. Add fruit and gently mix. Garnish with sunflower seeds and serve with fresh mint.

Serves 2.

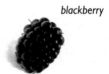

blackberry

Lychee is fast becoming available in supermarkets and is always found in Asian food markets. It has a rough reddish-brown skin, which peels away easily from the succulent, sweet, translucent fruit, and is high in B and C vitamins.

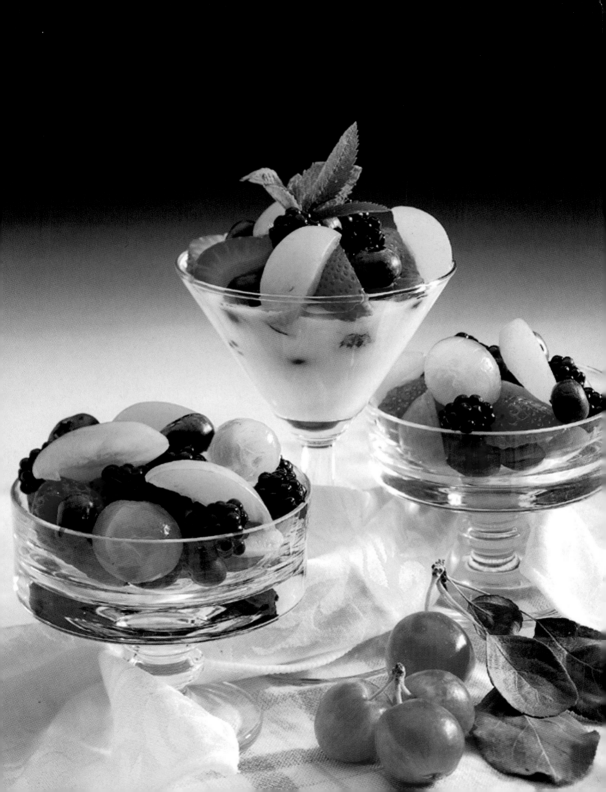

Blueberry Cornbread

Blueberries contain vitamins A, C, and B-complex, an abundance of iron, and most importantly for heart health, anthocyanin flavonoids, which are powerful antioxidants and help improve circulation.

2 cups (500 ml) **cornmeal**

1 cup (250 ml) **whole wheat flour, sifted twice**

3 (15 ml) **tsp baking powder**

1 ½ tsp (8 ml) **sea salt**

¼ cup (60 ml) **Sucanat or Rapadura**

1 ¼ cups (310 ml) **milk**

3 free-range eggs, beaten

¼ cup (60 ml) **butter, melted**

1 ½ cups blueberries

Preheat the oven to 375°F (190°C). Grease a 10" (25 cm) ovenproof cast-iron skillet or a loaf pan with 1 tablespoon of butter.

In a large bowl, combine cornmeal, flour, baking powder, salt, and Sucanat. Stir in milk, eggs, and butter, mixing until the dry ingredients are just moistened; add the blueberries.

Pour the batter into the skillet or loaf pan; bake for 20 to 25 minutes or until a toothpick inserted in the centre comes out clean.

Makes 1 loaf.

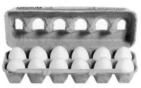

free-range eggs

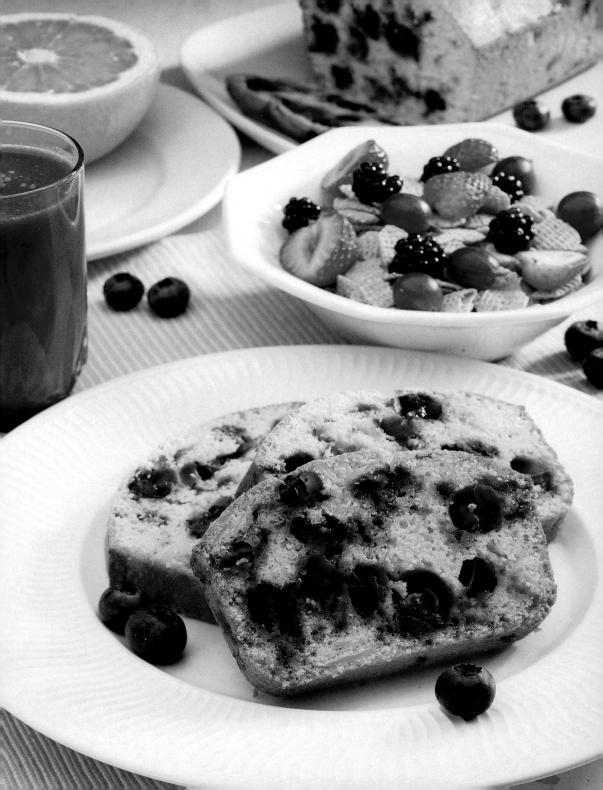

Arugula-Berry Salad

Fresh fruits and vegetables provide the flavonoids, enzymes, vitamins, and minerals needed for a well-oxygenated, healthy heart. The flavours in this salad come from around the world. Arugula comes from Italy, teardrop tomatoes from South America, sesame from the Far East, apple cider from France, and the berries are local. Altogether, the taste as well as the health benefits are fantastic wherever you are.

2 cups (500 ml) **arugula**

1 cup (250 ml) **mixed berries such as strawberries, blackberries, blueberries**

1 ½ cups (375 ml) **yam, cut matchstick-size**

1 cup (250 ml) **chayote squash, cut matchstick-size**

1 cup (250 ml) **teardrop tomatoes**

Sesame seeds, for garnish (optional)

Sesame-Apple Cider Dressing:

¼ cup (60 ml) **toasted sesame oil**

¼ cup (60 ml) **apple cider**

1 Tbsp (15 ml) **rice wine vinegar**

1 tsp (5 ml) **fresh lemon juice**

1 tsp (5 ml) **honey**

In a large bowl, whisk together all dressing ingredients. Add vegetables and fruit; toss well. Sprinkle with sesame seeds and serve.

Serves 2.

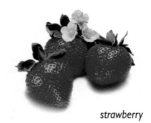

strawberry

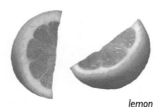

lemon

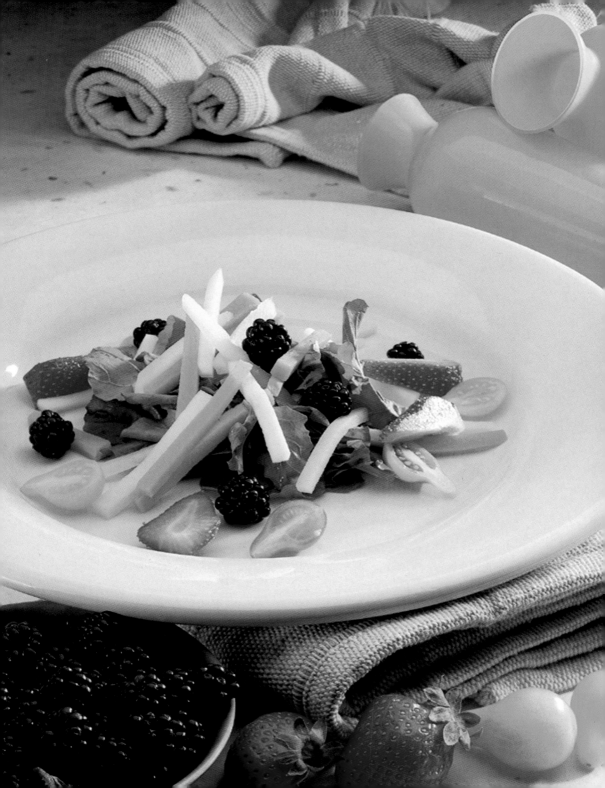

Coleslaw with Gooseberries and Figs

When people say "easy does it," they must be thinking of this quick recipe. You can shred all the vegetables and place them in the fridge, then, when you feel like having a nice coleslaw, you have it ready for a surprise meal without working hard for it. Besides the ease, it's also good for your heart. The vegetables and gooseberries provide vitamin C to protect artery walls and lower cholesterol while figs are rich in magnesium, which helps regulate heart activity.

1 cup (250 ml) **carrots, julienned**

1 ½ cups (375 ml) **Savoy cabbage, julienned**

1 cup (250 ml) **red onion, julienned**

1 cup (250 ml) **gooseberries**

2 fresh figs, sliced in thin wedges

Dressing:

1 ripe banana, mashed

¼ cup (60 ml) **extra-virgin olive oil**

2 Tbsp (30 ml) **sour cream**

1 tsp (5 ml) **fresh lime juice**

1 tsp (5 ml) **maple syrup**

1 tsp (5 ml) **fresh tarragon, chopped**

Mix together dressing ingredients in a blender. In a large bowl, combine carrots, cabbage, onion, and gooseberries then toss thoroughly with the dressing. Place salad onto plates, garnish with fresh figs, and serve.

Serves 2.

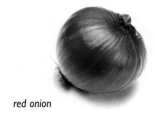

red onion

Did you know banana is actually a type of berry? I also recommend substituting gooseberries with loganberries or sun dried cranberries.

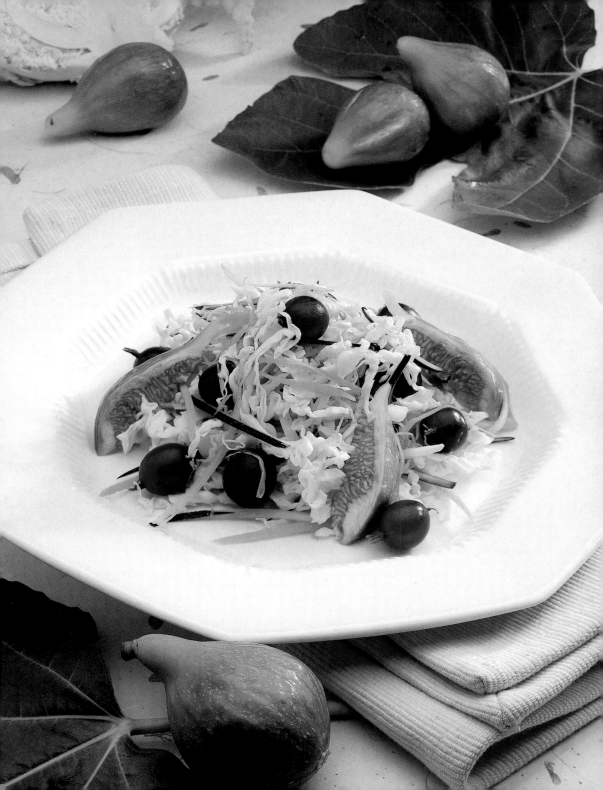

Marvelous Cranberry Muffins

Muffins are a treat and with this recipe, chalk full of cranberries, they are a nutritious treat! The entire family will enjoy them.

1 Tbsp (30 ml) **organic butter**

2 cups (500 ml) **whole wheat flour**

½ cup (125 ml) **natural cane sugar crystals**

5 tsp (25 ml) **baking powder**

½ tsp sea salt

¾ cup (300 ml) **natural, organic milk**

⅓ cup (100 ml) **unprocessed coconut oil**

1 free-range egg, beaten

1 cup (250 ml) **sun-dried cranberries**

¼ cup (60 ml) **crumbled hazelnuts**

Heat oven to 400° F (200° C). Grease 12 muffin cups (bottom only) with butter or line with paper baking cups. In medium bowl, combine flour, sugar crystals, baking powder, and sea salt; mix well. In another bowl combine milk, oil, and egg. Add mixture to dry ingredients. Stir until dry ingredients are slightly moistened (batter will be lumpy). Add cranberries and hazelnuts; mix well.

Fill muffin cups ⅔ full. Bake for 20 to 25 minutes or until toothpick inserted in center comes out clean. Cool for 1 minute before removing from pan.

Yields 12 muffins.

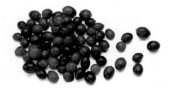

cranberries

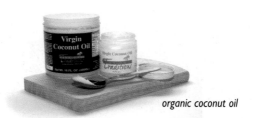

organic coconut oil

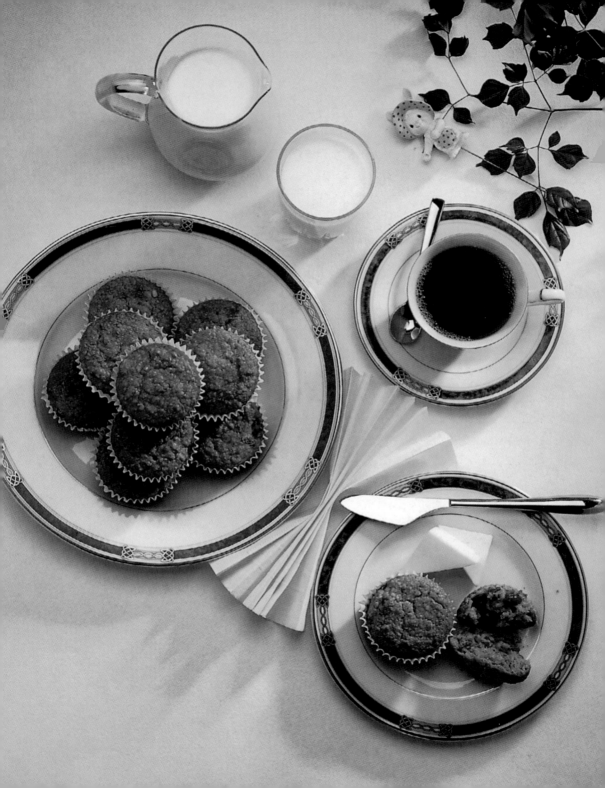

Oat-Banana Dumplings
with Blueberry Compote

The oats provide vitamin E to increase oxygen supply to the heart and improve heart muscle function; bananas supply potassium, which works with calcium and magnesium to control blood pressure and heart rhythm; pecans give you heart-healthy essential fatty acids; and, of course, the blueberries give you the all-important flavonoids.

Dumplings:

2 medium-ripe bananas, mashed with a fork

⅓ **cup** (80 ml) **rolled oats**

⅓ **cup** (80 ml) **pecans, roasted and freshly ground**

Pinch ground cinnamon

Pinch ground cloves

1 package round won ton wraps

2 Tbsp (30 ml) **butter**

Compote:

2 cups (500 ml) **blueberries**

1 Tbsp (15 ml) **maple syrup**

1 tsp (5 ml) **lime juice**

a pinch ground cardamom

In a bowl, combine banana, oats, pecans, and spices. Lay won ton wraps on a dry surface. Place 1 teaspoon of filling in the middle of each circle and brush the edges with a wet pastry brush. Fold the circle in a half-moon shape and press the edges together. (You can also shape the dumplings in a dumpling maker form.)

Bring a large pot of salted water to a boil. Drop the dumplings into the water and cook for 1 minute or until they float to the surface.

Scoop out the dumplings and drain thoroughly. Melt butter in a pan, add dumplings, and toss well.

In the meantime, mix all sauce ingredients together in another pan and toss on low heat until slightly warm and the juice comes out.

Place dumplings onto plates, pour the sauce over top and serve.

Serves 2.

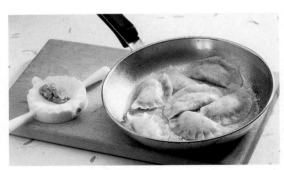

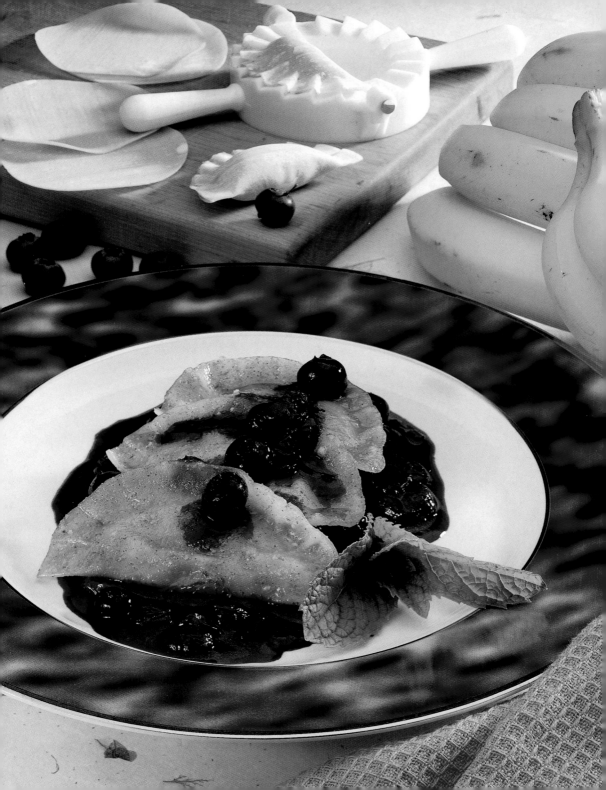

Blueberry-Yogurt
Timbale with Berry Sauce

Blueberry truly is a healing food that promotes circulation and strengthens the heart. Better yet, this wonderful berry is delicious and a pleasure to eat.

Timbale:

2 cups (500 ml)
  natural yogurt

1 cup (250 ml) **blueberries**

3 tsp (5 ml) **agar agar**

¼ cup (60 ml) **water**

1 ½ cups (375 ml) **cream**

½ cup (125 ml) **Sucanat**
  or Rapadura

1 tsp (5 ml) **vanilla extract**

Fresh mint leaves,
  for garnish

Sauce:

2 Tbsp (30 ml) **honey**

1 Tbsp (15 ml) **butter**

¾ cup (185 ml) **mixed**
  berries such as
  strawberries,
  blueberries, and
  blackberries

1 tsp (5 ml) **lime juice**

Rind of organic lime
  or lemon

To prepare the timbale, bring water to a boil in a small saucepan then add agar agar and stir until dissolved. In another saucepan, combine the cream and Sucanat, then cook over medium heat, stirring, for 5 minutes or until the Sucanat dissolves. Remove from heat then add the agar agar and mix thoroughly. Transfer the mixture into a bowl. Let cool for about 5 minutes, then whisk in the yogurt and vanilla; mix well. Stir in blueberries.

Rinse a 1-quart (1-liter) mold or individual molds with cold water then shake off excess water. Pour in the blueberry-yogurt mixture; place in the refrigerator, and chill for 2 to 3 hours.

Run the warm blade of a knife around the edge of the mold. Invert the mold and tap on it to loosen the blueberry-yogurt cream.

To make the sauce, heat honey and butter in a saucepan until melted. Stir in berries, lime juice, and rind; heat for 5 minutes.

Place blueberry-yogurt timbale onto plates, pour the warm sauce over top, garnish with mint and serve.

Serves 6.

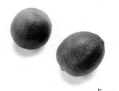

limes

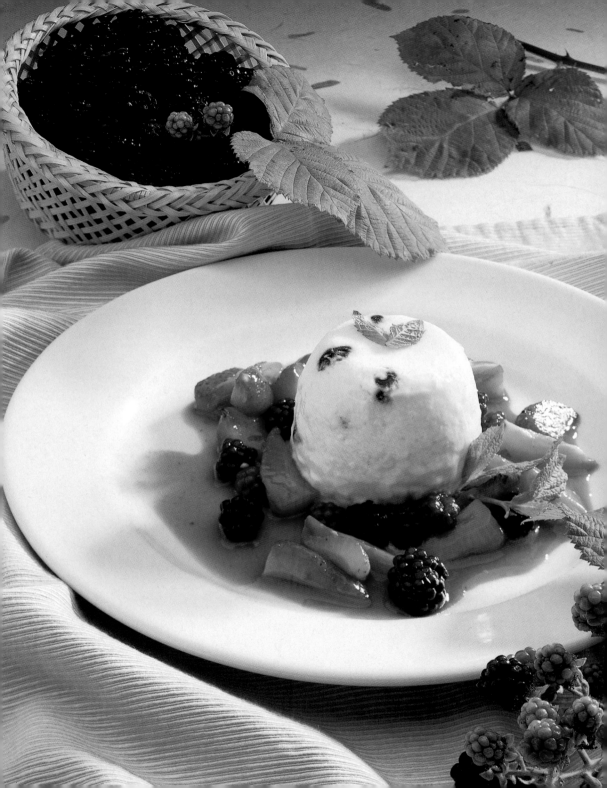

Three-Fruit Clafouti

Clafouti comes from southern France and was created to use up the bounty of the annual harvest. You'll be happy to know that this dish is not only eaten as dessert but as a meal. Don't forget the almonds–they're rich in essential fatty acids and vitamin E, which work together to lower cholesterol levels and keep the heart supplied with sufficient oxygen.

4 free-range eggs

⅓ cup (80 ml) **lavender honey**

1 vanilla bean, split in half or 1 tbsp (15 ml) **vanilla extract**

2 tbsp (30 ml) **butter, melted + 1 tbsp** (15 ml), **to grease pan**

⅔ cups (160 ml) **whole wheat flour, sifted twice**

1 ½ cups (375 ml) **whole milk**

1 lb (500 g) **mixed berries such as blueberries, cherries, blackberries**

½ cup (125 ml) **Sucanat or Rapadura**

½ cup (125 ml) **sliced almonds, toasted**

Confection Rapadura, for garnish

Preheat the oven to 350°F (180°C). Grease a 13"(33 cm) long baking dish with butter.

In a mixing bowl, whisk together the eggs and honey. Scrape the insides of the vanilla bean and add the pulp to the egg mixture (or add vanilla extract). Stir in the butter and flour then whisk in the milk to form a smooth batter.

In another mixing bowl, toss the berries with the Sucanat. Place the berries in the baking dish then pour the batter over top. Bake in the oven for 40 to 45 minutes or until the cake is sponge-like. Remove from the oven and cool for 5 minutes before serving.

Garnish with almonds, sprinkle with Rapadura, and serve warm with vanilla ice cream.

Serves 6 to 8.

Lavender Honey
Look for lavender honey in your local health food store, or you can easily make it at home. Boil 2 cups (500 ml) of fresh chopped lavender leaves and flowers in 1 cup (500 ml) of water until liquid is reduced to 1/4 cup (60 ml). Add to 2 cups (500 ml) of honey, mix well and use any time.

Baking Tip
Place a bowl of cold water in the oven in order to circulate the heat at an even temperature and keep the cake moist.

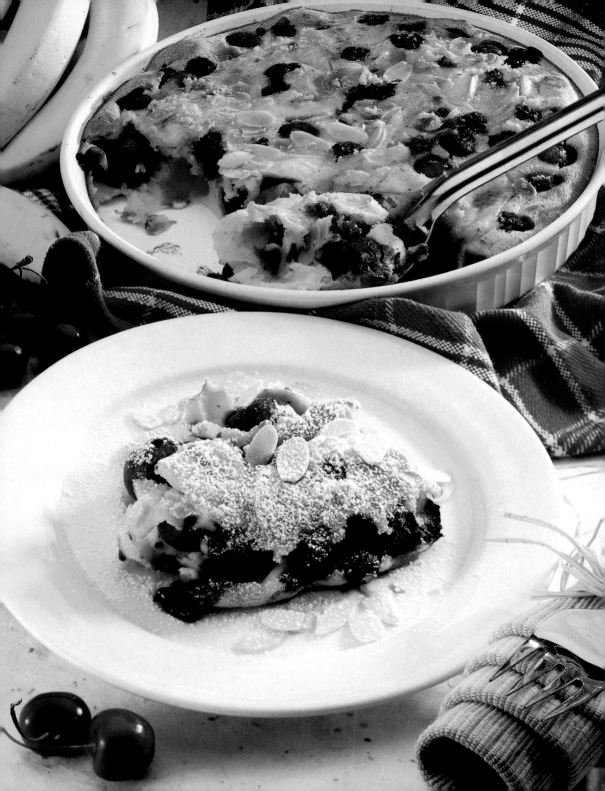

Cholesterol-Buster Flax seed Parfait (Christel's Rumpelstilskin)

This recipe can be served as breakfast, as dessert or late night snack. In any case, it is easily digested, helps for a good night's sleep, and keeps the intestines healthy and in good order. Flaxseeds have proven cholesterol lowering effects. Taking 50g of flax seed/day can bring a 9.8-percent reduction in LDL cholesterol and 19.8-percent reduction in Lipoprotein(a) (Lp(a)) within three weeks. For this purpose, flax seeds must be ground up first, because if they are eaten whole they will not be digested and will pass right through the digestive tract.

I6 Tbsp (240 ml) **flax seeds, preferably yellow/golden flax**

2 cups (500 ml) **milk**

2 Tbsp (30 ml) **ground hazelnuts**

1 banana

1 Tbsp (15 ml) **honey**

1 apple

1 orange, juice only

1 Tbsp (15 ml) **lemon juice**

Grind flax seeds in electric coffee grinder, boil milk, and stir in flax meal. Boil for 30 seconds, remove from heat, pour into a bowl and let cool. This substance looks like and has the consistency of a pudding, which is the base. Add to it the ground nuts, the banana mashed with a fork, honey, and the juice of the orange. Whisk vigorously or blend on lowest speed and serve in glass bowls or parfait glasses.

Optionally, when served as a dessert, top with whipping cream and blueberries, bilberries, cranberries, a strawberry or kiwi. Everyone, kids and adults alike, will enjoy this heavenly, delightful tasting concoction. Serves 4.

Varieties to the above delicacy:

To the base pudding you may add finely chopped dried and soaked fruits, strawberries, raspberries, blueberries, dates, figs, raisins, prunes, pineapples, etc.

Please visit *www.florahealth.com* for more information on the benefits of flax.

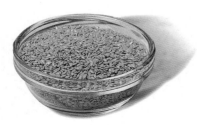

flax

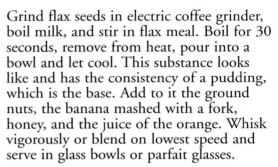

54

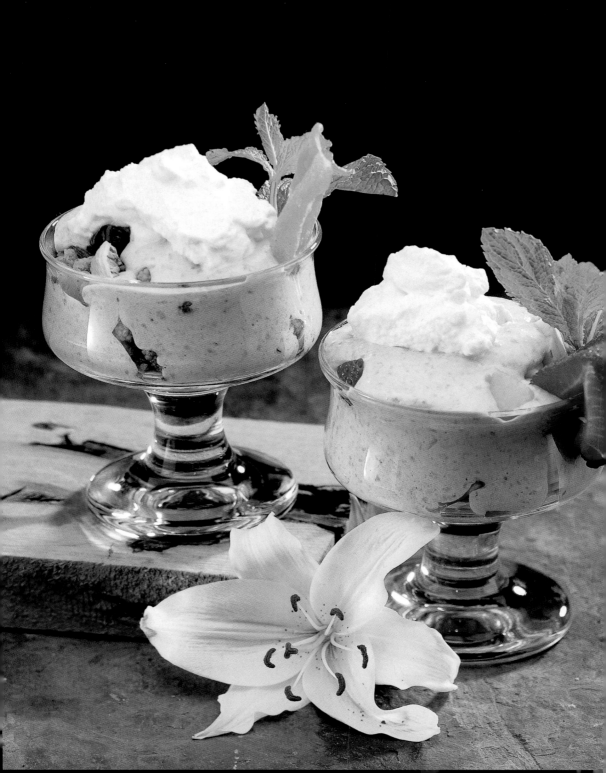

Sparkling Berry Punch

This refreshing punch is easy to make and is packed with a variety of heart-loving berries. Place it in the refrigerator and you can have it throughout a hot summer's day to keep you cool.

8 cups (2 litre) **cranberry juice**

6 cups (1 ½ litre) **sparkling mineral water**

2 cups (500 ml) **strawberries, hulled and quartered**

2 cups (500 ml) **cherries**

2 cups (500 ml) **gooseberries**

2 cups (500 ml) **raspberries**

2 cups (500 ml) **blueberries**

Fresh mint leaves and lemon slices, for garnish

Combine all ingredients in a large punch bowl. Garnish with mint and lemon slices and serve.

Fills 1 large punch bowl.

Variation: For special occasions, substitute champagne for the mineral water.

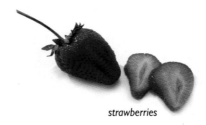

strawberries

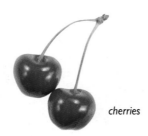

cherries

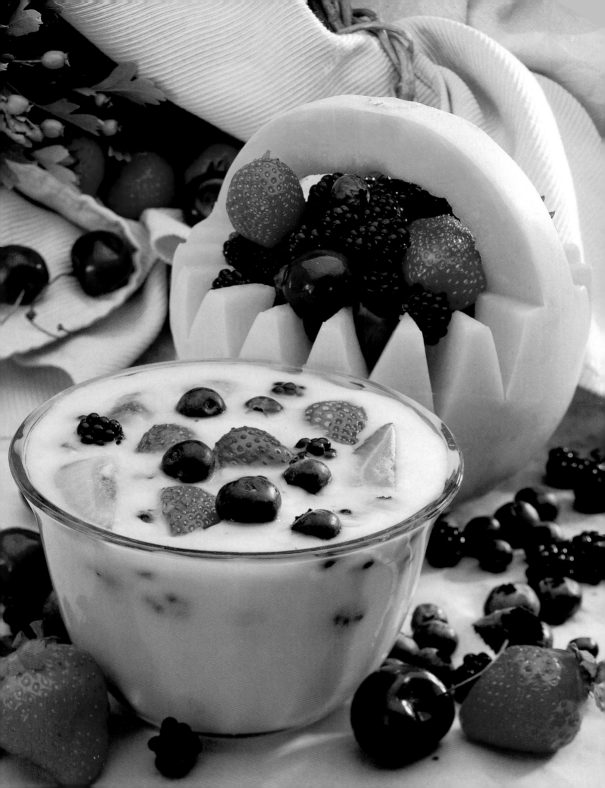

references

Allen, F.M. "Blueberry leaf extract: Physiologic and clinical properties in relation to carbohydrate metabolism." *Journal of the American Medical Association* 89 (1927): 1577-1581.

Ascherio, A. "Epidemiologic studies on dietary fats and coronary heart disease." *American Journal of Medicine* 113 (Dec. 2002) Suppl 9B: 9S-12S.

Assem, et al. "Inhibition of experimental asthma in man by a new drug (AH 7725) active when given by mouth." *British Medical Journal* 2 (1974): 93-95.

Aviram, M., et al. "Plasma lipid peroxidation: inhibited by drinking red wine but stimulated by white wine." *Harefuah* Vol.127, no.12 (1994): 517-520, 575-6.

Avorn J., et al. "Reduction of bacteriuria and pyuria after ingestion of cranberry juice" *Journal of the American Medical Association* 271 (1994): 751-754.

Bagchi D., et al. "Molecular mechanisms of cardioprotection by a novel grape seed proanthocyanidin extract." *Mutation Research* 523-524: (2003 Feb-Mar) 87-97.

—. "Benefits of resveratrol in women's health." *Drug Experimental & Clinical Research* 27(5-6): 233-48: (2001)

Bettini, V., et al. "Effects of Vaccinium myrtillus anthocyanosides on vascular smooth muscle." *Fitoterapia* 55 (1984): 265-272.

—. "Inhibition by Vaccinium myrtillus anthocyanosides of barium-induced contractions in segments of internal thoracic vein." *Fitoterapia* 55 (1984): 323-327.

—. "Mechanical responses of isolated coronary arteries to barium in the presence of Vaccinium myrtillus anthocyanosides." *Fitoterapia* 56 (1985): 3-10.

Blaszo, G. "Oedemia-inhibiting effects of procyanidin. "*Acta. Physiologica Academiae Hungaricea, Tomus.* "Vol. 65, no. 2 (1980): 235-240.

Bonanni, R. and G. Molinelli. "Clinical study of the action of myrtillin alone or associated with beta-carotene on normal subjects and on patients with degenerative changes of the fundus oculi." *Atti Accad Fisiocrit Siena [Med Fis]* Vol. 17, no. 2 (1968): 1470-1488.

Boniface, R. et al. "Pharmacological properties of myrtillus anthocyanosides: Correlation with results of treatment of diabetic microangiopathy." *Studies in Organic Chemistry* 23 (1986): 293-301.

Bottecchia, D., et al. "Preliminary report on the inhibitory effect of Vaccinium myrtillus anthocyanosides on platelet aggregation and clot retraction." *Fitoterapia* 48 (1987): 3-8.

Bravetti, G. "Preventive medical treatment of senile cataract with vitamin E and anthocyanosides: clinical evaluation." *Ann Ottalmol Clin Ocul* 115 (1989): 109.

Carper, J. *Food Your Miracle Medicine.* New York: Harper-Collins, (1993).

—. "*Miracle Cures.*" New York: HarperCollins (1997).

—."*Stop Aging Now.*" New York HarperCollins (1995).

Caselli, L. "Clinical and electroretinographic study on activity of anthocyanosides." *Arch Med Int.* 37 (1985): 29-35.

Colombo, D. and R. Bescovini. "Controlled trial of anthocyanosides from Vaccinium myrtillus in primary dysmenorrhea." *G Ital Obstet Ginecol.* 7 (1985): 1033-1038.

Cunnane, S. A., et al. "A Controlled Trial of Defatted Flax Seed in Hyperlipidemia." *Proceedings of the 56th Meeting of the Flax Institute of the United States.* (March 20-22, 1966): Fargo, ND.

Davies, MJ, et al., Black tea consumption reduces total and LDL cholesterol in mildly hypercholesterolemic adults. *Journal of Nutrition* 133 (10): (2003 Oct) 3298S-3302S.

de Lorgeril M, et al. "Mediterranean alpha-linolenic acid-rich diet in secondary prevention of coronary heart disease." *Lancet* 343(8911): (1994 Jun 11): 1454-9.

Demrow HS, et al. "Administration of wine and grape juice inhibits in vivo platelet activity and thrombosis in stenosed canine coronary arteries." *Circulation* 91(4): (1995 Feb 15): 1182-8.

Detre Z, et al. "Studies on vascular permeability in hypertension: action of anthocyanosides." *Clinical & Physiological Biochemstry.* 4(2): (1986): 143-9.

Diamond, Suzanne M. "*Herb and Supplement Encyclopedia.*" Published by Florahealth.com website. http://www.florahealth.com/flora/home/canada/healthinformation/encyclopedias/_main.asp.

Djousse, L., et al. "National Heart, Lung, and Blood Institute Family Heart Study. 2003. Dietary linolenic acid and carotid atherosclerosis. *American Journal of Clinical Nutrition.* 77(4): (2003 Apr): 819-25.

Erasmus, Udo. *Fats that Heal, Fats that Kill.* Burnaby, B.C.: Alive Publishing (1993): pp. 1-456.

Fokina, GI., et al. "Experimental phytotherapy of tick-borne encephalitis." *Voprosy Virusologii.* Vol. 36, no. 1 (1991): 18-21.

Folts, JD. "Potential health benefits from the flavonoids in grape products on vascular disease." *Advanced Exp Med Biol*. 505: (2002): 95-111.

–. "A perspective on the potential problems with aspirin as an antithrombotic agent: a comparison of studies in an animal model with clinical trials." *Journal of the American College of Cardiology* 33(2): (1999 Feb): 295-303.

Freedman, JE, et al. "Select flavonoids and whole juice from purple grapes inhibit platelet function and enhance nitric oxide release." *Circulation* 103(23): (2001 Jun 12): 2792-8.

Gloria, E. and A. Perla. "Activity of anthocyanosides on absolute visual threshold." *Annals Ottalm Clin Ocul*. 92 (1966): 595-605.

Grismond, GL "Treatment of pregnancy-induced phlebopathies." *Minerva Ginecol*. 33 (1981): 221-230.

Howell, A B., et al. "Inhibition of the adherence of p-fimbriated escherichia coli to uroepithelial-cell surfaces by proanthocyanidin extracts from cranberries." *New England Journal of Medicine* Vol. 339, no. 15 (1998): 1085-86.

Jenkins, DJ, et al. "Dose response of almonds on coronary heart disease risk factors: blood lipids, oxidized low-density lipoproteins, lipoprotein(a), homocysteine, and pulmonary nitric oxide: a randomized, controlled, crossover trial." *Circulation* 106(11): (2002 Sep 10): 1327-32.

Katsube, N, et al. "Induction of apoptosis in cancer cells by Bilberry (*Vaccinium myrtillus*) and the anthocyanins". *J Agric Food Chem* 51(1): (2003 Jan 1): 68-75.

Keevil, JG, et al. "Grape juice, but not orange juice or grapefruit juice, inhibits human platelet aggregation." *Journal of Nutrition* 130(1): (2000 Jan): 53-6.

Kelly, JP et al. "Risk of aspirin-associated major upper gastrointestinal bleeding with enteric-coated or buffered product." *Lancet* 348 (1996): 1413-16.

Lietti, et al. "Studies on Vaccinium myrtillus anthocyanosides. I. Vasoprotective and antiinflammatory activity." *Arzneimittelforschung* Vol. 26, no. 5 (1976): 829-832.

Logan, AC, Wong, C. "Chronic fatigue syndrome: oxidative stress and dietary modifications." *Alternative Medicine Review* : 6(5): (2001 Oct): 450-9.

Lovejoy, JC. "The influence of dietary fat on insulin resistance." *Curr Diab Rep* 2(5): (2002 Oct): 435-40.

Magistretti, et al. "Antiulcer activity of an anthocyanidin from Vaccinium." *Arzneimittelforschung* 38 (1988): 686-690.

Masquelier, J. "Stabilisation du collagen par les oligomeres procyanidoliques." *Acta Therap.* 7 (1981): 101-105.

Mazza, G. and Miniati, E. *"Anthocyanins in Fruits, Vegetables and Grains"*. Boca Raton, FL: CRC Press (1993).

Mian, A. et al. "Anthocyanosides and the walls of microvessels: further aspects of the mechanism of action of their protective effect in syndromes due to abnormal capillary fragility." *Minerva Medica* Vol. 68, no. 52 (1977): 3565-3581.

Murray, MT. "Bilberry (Vaccinium myrtillus)." *American Journal of Natural Medicine* Vol. 4, no. 1 (1997): 18-22.

Ofek, I., et al. "Anti-escherichia coli adhesion activity of cranberry and blueberry juices." *New England Journal of Medicine* Vol. 324, no. 22 (1991): 1599.

Passwater, R. A. "Sun damage, skin and Pycnogenol: An interview with Dr. Antti Arstila." *Whole Foods*, (August 1994).

Politzer, M. "Experiences in the treatment of progressive myopia." *Klinische Monatsblätter für Augenheilkunde*. Vol. 171, no. 4 (1977): 616-9.

Reaven, GM. "The role of insulin resistance and hyperinsulinemia in coronary heart disease." *Metabolism* 41 (1992): 16-19.

Reed, J. "Cranberry flavonoids, atherosclerosis and cardiovascular health." *Critical Review of Food Science Nutrition* 42(3 Suppl): (2002): 301-16.

Rein, D. et al., "Cocoa inhibits platelet activation and function." *American Journal of Clinical Nutrition* 72(1): 2000 Jul; 30-5.

Robert, L. "The effect of procyanidolic oligomers on vascular permeability." *Pathologie Biologie*. Vol. 3, (1990): 608-616.

Rusniyak, S. and A. Szent-Gyorgi. "Vitamin P: flavonoids as vitamins." *Nature* 138 (1936): 27.

Sala, D. et al. "Effect of anthocyanosides on visual performances at low illumination". *Minerva Oftalmologic* 21 (1979): 283-285.

Sato, M, et al. "Cardioprotective effects of grape seed proanthocyanidin against ischemic reperfusion injury." *Journal of Molecular and Cellular Cardiology*. 31(6): (1999 Jun): 1289-97.

Terrasse, J. and S. Moinade. "Premiers resultats obtenus avec un nouveau facteur vitaminique P 'les anthocyanosides' extraits du Vaccinium myrtillus." *Presse Medicale* 72 (1964): 397-400.

Vanderhaeghe, LR. and PJD. Bouic. *The Immune System Cure: Nature's Way to Supper-Powered Health*. (Scarborough, ON: Prentice-Hall, 2000).

von Eiff, M., et al. "Examination of the pharmaceutical quality, safety and therapeutic effects of a Crataegus/Passiflora-extract." Thesis, Universität Basel, 1994.

–. "Hawthorn/passion flower extract and improvement in physical exercise capacity of patients with dyspnoea class II of the NYHA functional classification." *Acta Therapeutica*. 20(1-2): (1994): 47-66.

Wegmann, R., et al. "Effects of anthocyanosides on photoreceptors. Cytoenzymatic aspects." *Annals of Histochemistry* 14 (1969): 237-256.

Werbach, MR., and MT Murray. *Botanical Influences on Illness*. (Tarzana, CA: Third Line Press: 1991).

Willaman, JJ. "Some biological effects of flavonoids." *Journal of the American Pharmaceutical Association* 44 (1955): 404-407.

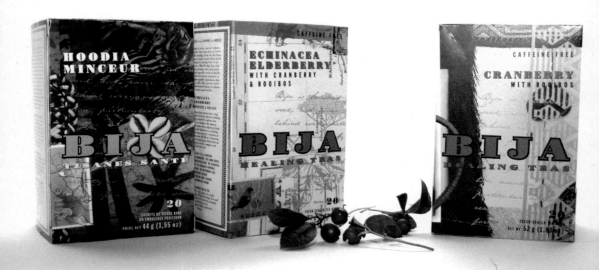